Instructor's Resource Manual and Testbank
to Accompany Rosdahl & Kowalski's

Textbook of Basic Nursing

EIGHTH EDITION

Lisa Wehner, RN, MS, CCRN, FNP

Associate Professor of Nursing
State University of New York at Delhi
Delhi, New York

LIPPINCOTT WILLIAMS & WILKINS
A **Wolters Kluwer** Company

Philadelphia • Baltimore • New York • London
Buenos Aires • Hong Kong • Sydney • Tokyo

Managing Editor: Doris S. Wray
Senior Production Editor: Rosanne Hallowell
Senior Production Manager: Helen Ewan
Managing Editor / Production: Erika Kors
Manufacturing Manager: William Alberti
Compositor: Lippincott Williams & Wilkins
Printer: Victor Graphics

ISBN: 0-7817-3431-2

Any procedure or practice described in this book should be applied by the health care practitioner under appropriate supervision in accordance with professional standards of care used with regard to the unique circumstances that apply in each practice situation. Care has been taken to confirm the accuracy of information presented and to describe generally accepted practices. However, the authors, editors, and publisher cannot accept any responsibility for errors or omissions or for any consequences from application of the information in this book and make no warranty, express or implied, with respect to the contents of the book.

Contents

CHAPTER 1

The Origins of Nursing

LEARNING OBJECTIVES

1. Describe events in ancient and medieval times that influenced the development of contemporary nursing.

2. Discuss Florence Nightingale's influence on modern nursing practice.

3. List at least 10 of Florence Nightingale's nursing principles that are still practiced today.

4. Identify important individuals who contributed to the development of nursing in the United States.

5. Name some pioneer nursing schools in the United States.

6. List important milestones in the history of practical nursing education.

7. Explain developments in nursing related to war.

8. Discuss current trends that are expected to influence the nursing profession into the 21st century.

9. Describe the importance of nursing insignia, uniforms, and the nursing school pin.

NEW TERMINOLOGY

caduceus	insignia
Hippocratic oath	Nightingale lamp
holistic healthcare	

KEY POINTS

- Medicine men and women and religious orders cared for the sick in early times.
- Florence Nightingale contributed a great deal to the development of contemporary nursing.
- Establishment of nursing schools in the United States began in the late 19th century.
- The first practical nursing school in the United States opened in 1892 in New York.

- Nursing during the First and Second World Wars contributed to the profession's and to women's evolving roles in society.
- Many current societal and healthcare trends are influencing the nursing profession, including higher levels of client acuity in hospital settings, more community-based care, technological advances, changing lifestyles, greater life expectancy, changing nursing education, and more nursing autonomy.
- Nursing insignia, such as those found on nursing school pins, often symbolize nursing's history and heritage.

■ Teaching–Learning Strategies

CLASSROOM

1. Ask the students to define the following terms or abbreviations:

AIDS	NCLEX
AJN	NLN
ANA	RN
AMA	VNS
HOSA	YMCA
ICN	YWCA
LPN	community-based care
LVN	holistic healthcare
NAPNES	insignia

Write the students' responses on the chalkboard or on an overhead transparency.

2. Conduct a brief discussion about the origins of the practical nursing program in which the students are enrolled. Ask the director of the nursing program to offer brief remarks to the students in the class. Ask a nurse who has retired from the nursing profession to visit the class and share information about her nursing duties from the past.

3. Before the class, write the names of significant individuals and/or dates in nursing on 3 × 5

index cards. In the classroom, divide students into pairs and give each group an index card. Ask students to identify the accomplishments of the person or to identify the significance of the particular date on the index card. Ask students to share their findings with the class.

4. Before the class, using an overhead transparency, list the principles of nursing as outlined by Florence Nightingale. Ask students to identify which principles should still exist today.

5. Ask students to identify how the changing roles of women in society helped contribute to the changing role of nursing. Conduct a brief discussion about advanced practice roles in nursing (e.g., family nurse practitioners, nurse midwives).

6. During the class, conduct a discussion about the current trends in nursing. Ask students to identify how these trends might affect their practice.

7. If possible, locate several nursing school pins. Pass these pins around so students can look at them. Ask students to identify the various symbols on the pins.

CLINICAL

1. Take students on a brief tour of a hospital unit that they will be assigned to for their clinical experience. Ask the students to record their observations about the unit, the staff, and the patients. Ask students to observe whether any of the nurses are wearing insignia, such as a school pin. Meet with the students after the tour and ask them to share their observations.

2. Ask students to interview a nurse about the history of nursing and significant nursing leaders. Ask the students to write a one- to two-page paper about their interview. Ask students to share the interview in a classroom setting.

3. Assign a small group of students to a clinical setting that uses an advanced practice nurse. Ask the students to record their observations about the role of the advance practice nurse. Ask the students to share their findings with the rest of the class.

CHAPTER 2

Beginning Your Nursing Career

LEARNING OBJECTIVES

1. Compare the education and level of practice between registered and practical nurses.

2. Explain the various types of educational programs that lead to licensure.

3. Identify at least one of the standards of the National Federation of Licensed Practical Nurses in relationship to each of the following: education, legal status, and practice.

4. Differentiate between permissive and mandatory licensure.

5. Discuss the reasons for a nurse to seek licensure.

6. Identify the importance of the nurse's pledge.

7. Explain the importance of nursing theory and how a theoretical framework helps nurses in their learning, understanding, and practice.

8. List the roles of today's nurse, briefly explaining each one.

9. Discuss the importance of nurses projecting a professional image.

10. Describe nursing organizations, their membership requirements, and benefits.

NEW TERMINOLOGY

accreditation	nurse practice act
advanced practice nurse	permissive licensure
approval	practical nurses
licensure	registered nurses
mandatory licensure	theoretical framework

KEY POINTS

- Differences exist in the education and level of nursing practice between RNs and PNs.
- Several types of nursing education lead to licensure as a registered nurse or as a practical/vocational nurse.

- Only graduates of state-, commonwealth-, territory-, or province-approved schools of nursing are eligible to write the licensure examination.
- Most states have mandatory licensure laws for nurses. Nurse licensure is available in all states, territories, and Canadian provinces.
- Nurses promise to practice ethically when they recite pledges at graduation.
- Many nursing programs base their curricula on nursing theories. These theoretical frameworks provide reasons and purposes for nursing actions.
- The nurse assumes many roles. Many responsibilities accompany the title of "nurse."
- Projecting a professional image is important. Such an image helps nurses to properly represent their school, place of employment, and the healthcare industry. Moreover, it serves to protect and maintain safety for clients and nurses.
- Nursing organizations set standards of practice for RNs and LPNs. A primary nursing responsibility is to be familiar with these standards.
- Nursing organizations assist in continuing education and collective bargaining. In addition, they offer a forum for discussion of nursing issues with peers.

■ Teaching–Learning Strategies

CLASSROOM

1. Ask the students to define the following terms and abbreviations:

AALPN	accreditation
AD	approval
ANCC	advanced practice nurse
CAN	licensure
E-mail	NFLPN
INC	permissive licensure
NCLEX-PN	theoretical framework
NLN-CHAP	mandatory licensure
UAP	

2. Before the class, divide an overhead transparency into two vertical columns. On one side of the transparency list the three types of programs that lead to an RN licensure. On the other side of the transparency, list the types of programs that lead to LPN or LVN licensure. Ask students to discuss the differences in the various programs.

3. On an overhead transparency, identify the standards of practice for LPNs and LVNs. Ask students to provide examples of nursing activities for each standard.

4. Review the nursing practice standards for the LPN/LVN. Ask students to provide examples of nursing activities for each standard.

5. Ask students to discuss the differences between mandatory and permissive licensure requirements. Ask the students if the state they live in has a mandatory or permissive licensure requirement.

6. On an overhead transparency, list the following theorists: Florence Nightingale, Virginia Henderson, Dorothea Orem, Sister Callista Roy, and Betty Neuman. Ask students to identify the model and the concepts for each theorist. Provide students with examples of nursing activities for each of the theorists (e.g., Orem's Self-Care Model—when a nurse helps a client to perform a daily bath).

7. List the following nursing roles on an overhead transparency or the chalkboard: care provider, communicator, teacher, advocate, leader, and team member. Ask the students to identify nursing activities that would fall under each category.

8. Ask the students about their impressions of nurses with whom they have had contact. Ask them to share their impressions with the class. Ask students what influences the media have had on images of nursing (e.g., television soap operas, movies, etc.). Discuss the misconceptions or distorted images that individuals may have about nursing as a profession.

9. Ask a nurse who is actively involved in a nursing organization to visit the class and explain her activities. Open the class for discussion after the presentation.

10. Quiz the students at the end of the class.

CLINICAL

1. Ask students to interview a nurse and determine if the nurse is active in a professional nursing organization. Ask students to share their findings with the class.

2. Take a group of students to the clinical setting where they will have their clinical experiences. Ask the students to select one nurse to follow for a short time period. Ask the students to record the nurse's activities and categorize these activities into the various nursing roles. Ask the students to share their findings in class.

3. Arrange for a pair of students to visit an outpatient or community clinic. Ask the students to observe a nurse's activities and categorize these activities into the various nursing roles. Ask the students to share their findings in class.

Short Answer

1. The regulation by some states to make it illegal for a nurse to practice without a license is termed _____ licensure. (*Ans:* mandatory)

2. Licensure laws establish a minimum _____ of _____ for competence and practice. (*Ans:* level; requirements)

3. Sister Callista Roy is a nurse theorist associated with the model of _____. (*Ans:* adaptation)

4. A vocational organization designed specifically for students in secondary and postsecondary health occupation is ____. (*Ans:* Health Occupations Students of America)

5. When a nurse documents client care and the client's response the nurse is acting in the role of a _____. (*Ans:* communicator)

VOCABULARY DEVELOPMENT

Ask students to define the following terms:

1. Accreditation: voluntary activity by a school or program to ensure quality of education

2. Licensure: laws establishing a minimal level of requirements for competence

3. Advocate: nurses serve in this role to make sure that clients receive necessary care and intervention when necessary

4. Professional image: the image that the nurse projects to the public as a representative of the school/program and the nursing profession

CHAPTER 3

The Healthcare Delivery System

LEARNING OBJECTIVES

1. Discuss at least three trends and challenges of healthcare in the 21st century. Relate these changes to the needs of nurses, healthcare practitioners, and the consumers of healthcare (clients).

2. Define and discuss at least three differences between acute care and extended care facilities.

3. Identify at least two types of healthcare services provided in each type of healthcare facility.

4. Identify at least three services available to meet the healthcare needs of the community.

5. State at least two functions of a school nurse and an industrial nurse.

6. State at least two functions of the Joint Commission on Accreditation of Healthcare Organizations (JCAHO). Relate these functions to nursing standards of care.

7. Define the term *quality assurance* and state its function in healthcare facilities.

8. Explain the role of the client representative, advocate, or ombudsperson.

9. Describe at least six methods of payment for healthcare services.

10. Determine the role of complementary or holistic care in the delivery of healthcare.

11. Identify at least three negative impacts of consumer fraud on public wellness.

NEW TERMINOLOGY

acuity	incentive programs
capitation fee	managed care
case management	Medicaid
chain of command	Medicare
client	outcome-based care
complementary	patient
co-pay	prospective payment
holism	quality assurance
holistic healthcare	telehealth
home healthcare	third-party payment
hospice	

KEY POINTS

- Many changes in the healthcare system in the 21st century will bring new and unknown challenges for nurses.
- Types of healthcare facilities include hospitals, which now primarily treat people with acute conditions; extended care facilities, where care is given for a longer time; and community services, which include outpatient care, walk-in care, home healthcare, and care in schools and industries. Employment opportunities for nurses exist in all these areas.
- The JCAHO establishes quality and appropriate care standards.
- Many hospitals have established the position of client advocate (representative, ombudsperson) to help the client and family adapt to hospital stays.
- Third-party payment has been the method of payment for healthcare in the United States for a number of years. A variety of organizations provide this service.
- Complementary healthcare will play an increasing role in the healthcare delivery system of the United States in the future.
- Holism is a philosophy that views the "whole person."

■ Teaching–Learning Strategies

CLASSROOM

1. Ask the students to define the following terms or abbreviations:

CQI	SSDI
DRG	Medicaid
ECF	Medicare
HMO	co-pay
HPRDA	telehealth
ICF	wellness
HIS	holism
JCAHO	advocacy
OSHA	consumer fraud
PPO	client outcome-based care
RUG	unlicensed assistive personnel

   Write the students' responses on the chalkboard or on an overhead transparency.

2. Invite a nurse who is employed in a healthcare setting to describe changes that have occurred related to client care during the past few years. After the presentation, open the class for discussion.

3. Before class, obtain several "critical pathways" or nursing care paths from various healthcare settings. Pass them around during the class and ask students to compare and contrast the various paths. Explain to students the rationale for clinical pathways.

4. Before class, using an overhead transparency, list the healthcare problems facing the United States. Ask students to predict how these problems will affect nursing.

5. On an overhead transparency, outline a definition of "holistic healthcare." Ask students to describe nursing responsibilities in this type of healthcare.

6. List the various types of healthcare settings on the chalkboard or an overhead transparency. Ask students to indicate the type of setting in which they hope to be employed and their reasons for choosing that type of setting.

7. Briefly discuss standards of quality assurance. Ask students to identify definitions of these standards.

8. Before class, using an overhead transparency, outline the various methods of healthcare financing. Ask students to identify the impact of changes in third-party payment.

9. Briefly discuss "alternative healthcare providers" and ask students to share their experiences, if any, with these providers. Ask students to identify the potential problems associated with consumer fraud.

CLINICAL

1. Take a group of students to a healthcare setting. Ask the students to review client charts to determine the type of healthcare payment.

2. While at a healthcare setting, ask students to locate the policy manuals and review various procedures and policies.

3. Ask a client representative or advocate to speak to the group about roles in the particular healthcare setting. Follow the presentation with time for questions and answers.

4. Take a small group of students to a healthcare setting that has a physical therapy, rehabilitation, or occupational therapy department and take a brief tour. Ask students to share their observations with the class.

CHAPTER 4

Legal and Ethical Aspects of Nursing

LEARNING OBJECTIVES

1. Define the following medical–legal terms: crime, felony, misdemeanor, liability, tort, negligence, malpractice, assault, battery, informed consent, libel, and slander.

2. Discuss the concept of false imprisonment and relate the discussion to your daily nursing practice.

3. Explain at least three implications for nurses associated with the issues of abandonment of care, invasion of privacy, and confidentiality.

4. State at least five special healthcare issues and relate them to nursing.

5. Define and discuss the purpose of a Nurse Practice Act.

6. State at least four components of a Nurse Practice Act.

7. State at least three functions of a State Board of Nursing.

8. State the purpose of the NCLEX-PN.

9. State at least eight common sense precautions that nurses can take against lawsuits.

10. State at least two benefits and two limitations of the Good Samaritan Act.

11. Discuss at least four rationales for the concepts of professional boundaries.

12. Define and discuss the three major types of advance directives.

13. State three types of persons who are vulnerable to deficient or harmful care.

14. Differentiate between biological and brain death.

15. Define and discuss at least four ethical concepts that relate to nursing.

16. State at least three rights of healthcare clients and three responsibilities of healthcare clients.

NEW TERMINOLOGY

advance directive	Good Samaritan Act
assault	informed consent
assisted suicide	liability
battery	libel
brain death	malpractice
crime	misdemeanor
endorsement	negligence
ethics	Nurse Practice Act
euthanasia	slander
felony	tort

KEY POINTS

- You are legally and ethically bound to practice nursing within the rules and regulations of your Nursing Practice Act and within the laws of your state, territory, or province.
- Several types of advance directives allow individuals to plan ahead and to make decisions in advance about healthcare to be received if they become incapacitated.
- Individuals have the right to accept or to refuse treatment in most situations.
- You will encounter many ethical decisions in healthcare. Some of these require the assistance of an ethics committee.

■ Teaching–Learning Strategies

CLASSROOM

1. Ask the students to define the following terms and abbreviations:

AHA	malpractice tort
AMA	felony
CEU	euthanasia
CNS	misdemeanor
NAHC	slander
PSDA	fraud
UNOS	assault
ethics	assisted suicide
crime	advanced directives
negligence	informed consent

Write the students' responses on the chalkboard or on an overhead transparency.

2. Invite a nurse lawyer to visit the class and present legal aspects of nursing. After the presentation, open the class for discussion.

3. On an overhead transparency or chalkboard, write the terms liability, negligence, fraud, assault and battery, abandonment of care, libel, and slander. Ask students to define the terms and provide possible situations for each term. Conduct a brief discussion about ways that nurses and students can safeguard themselves.

4. Before class, obtain a blank institutional form for "informed consent." Pass the form around during the class and discuss issues related to informed consent.

5. Conduct a brief discussion in class about living wills and advance directives. Ask students to write their own "living wills" and share their writings in class.

6. Select several patient/client rights from the Patient's Bill of Rights. Ask students to discuss what each of these rights means to them.

7. Before class, on 3 × 5 index cards, write various case studies with ethical implications. This could include issues such as euthanasia, keeping a client on life support indefinitely, or other situations. Distribute the cards in class and ask students in pairs to outline what actions they would take in these situations.

CLINICAL

1. Take a small group of students to the clinical agency where they will have their clinical experiences. Ask the students to review charts of surgical clients and review the informed consents. Meet with the group and ask students to share their findings.

2. Ask a nurse who is a member of the institution's ethics committee to meet with a small group of students. Conduct a discussion about the functions of the ethics committee and open the presentation for discussion.

3. In the clinical setting, ask students to review the policy manuals related to ethical issues. Ask students to share their findings.

4. In a clinical setting, ask each student to interview a nurse about potential legal or ethical situations. Ask students to share their findings in clinical conference.

SUGGESTED RESOURCES

Ellis, J. R., & Hartley, C. L. (1997). *Nursing in today's world: Challenges, issues, and trends* (6th ed.). Philadelphia: Lippincott-Raven.
Ethics and economics: The rising cost of health care. [Videotape, 30 minutes]. (Available from Films for the Humanities and Sciences, P.O. Box 2053, Princeton, NJ 08543-2053; 800-257-5126; *www.films.com*)
Having the time of your life: Time management for students. (1997). [Videotape]. (Available from Nimco, Inc., P.O. Box 9, 102 Highway 81 North, Calhoun, KY 42327; 800-962-6662)
Joel, L. (1995). Your license to practice: Variations on a theme. *American Journal of Nursing, 95*(11), 7.
Nursing. (1994). [Videotape, 20 minutes]. (Available from Nimco, Inc., P.O. Box 9, 102 Highway 81 North, Calhoun, KY 42327; 800-962-6662)

CHAPTER 5

Basic Human Needs

LEARNING OBJECTIVES

1. Describe and discuss the hierarchy of needs from the simple to the complex as developed by Maslow.

2. State the rationale for regression from one level to another in the hierarchy.

3. List at least five physiologic needs of all people and animals.

4. List five examples of nursing activities that help an individual meet basic human needs.

5. List four examples of nursing activities that help an individual meet the needs of security and safety.

6. List two examples of nursing activities that help an individual obtain the goal of self-esteem.

7. List two examples of nursing activities that help an individual obtain the goal of self-actualization.

8. Address the basic and aesthetic needs of individuals who are homeless, have a terminal illness, or have lost their jobs and source of income.

9. Relate at least three community or societal needs to the hierarchy of needs of an individual.

NEW TERMINOLOGY

aesthetic needs	regression
hierarchy of needs	secondary needs
homeostasis	self-actualized
physiologic needs	self-esteem
primary needs	social needs
psychological needs	survival needs

KEY POINTS

- Physiologic needs drive all human beings and animals.
- Human needs are thought of in levels, known as a hierarchy.
- Psychological needs are at a higher level than physiologic needs.
- A person must meet lower level needs before he or she can address higher level needs.
- Illness or injury can interfere with a person's ability to meet needs.
- Illness or injury also can cause a person to regress to a lower level of functioning.
- Nursing can assist a person to meet needs or to eliminate potential threats to need satisfaction.
- Many factors, such as loss of income, illness, homelessness, and personal crises, threaten basic human needs.
- Health is a continually fluctuating and fluid state of physiologic and psychological well-being.
- Relationships with others, including family and the community, are higher level needs that can be addressed only after basic physiologic needs are met.

■ Teaching–Learning Strategies

CLASSROOM

1. Before class, using an overhead transparency, outline the pyramid of Maslow's Hierarchy of Human Needs. During the class, ask students to list various needs that would fall under each category.

2. Ask students to share their experiences related to their human needs. Ask students to describe a situation in which their basic needs had to be satisfied before other higher level needs could be met.

3. Ask students to discuss family and community needs. Conduct a discussion about various needs within a particular community and how healthcare influences these needs (e.g., immunization programs, health screening, drinking water safety).

CLINICAL

1. Take a small group of students to a hospital setting. Ask students to interview one client by focusing on how nurses have helped the client to meet his or her basic needs. Ask the students to share their findings during clinical conference.

2. Arrange for a small group of students to visit a homeless shelter. Ask students to interview a staff member about how the person assists the residents to meet their basic human needs.

3. Take a small group of students to a community outpatient clinic or public health clinic. Ask students to interview a nurse about the role of healthcare in meeting family or community needs. Ask students to share their findings with the larger group.

CHAPTER 6

Health and Wellness

LEARNING OBJECTIVES

1. State the World Health Organization's definition of health.

2. List five components of health and describe how each is attained.

3. Define and differentiate the terms *morbidity* and *mortality*.

4. Discuss at least four effects the financing of healthcare has on nursing.

5. State at least three preventative healthcare measures that have benefited American society.

6. Explain the wellness–illness continuum. Discuss the implications of acute and chronic illnesses as part of the continuum.

7. Relate the concept of wellness to Maslow's hierarchy of human needs.

8. Define and differentiate the terms *lifestyle factor* and *risk factor*.

9. State at least five lifestyle or risk factors that can directly affect health. Identify at least three nursing considerations for each factor.

10. List at least four sources of healthcare education and information.

11. Identify at least three health concerns of each of the following age groups: infants, children, adolescents and young adults, mature adults, and older adults. State at least four nursing implications related to each.

12. Identify at least nine categories of diseases and disorders that are deviations from wellness.

NEW TERMINOLOGY

acute illness	illness
benign	infection
carcinogenic	lifestyle factor
chronic illness	local
congenital disorders	malignant
contagious	metastasis
defense mechanisms	morbidity
disease	mortality
domestic violence	myocardial infarction
dysfunctional	neoplastic
elder abuse	organic disease
etiology	osteoporosis
functional disease	preterm birth
health	risk factor
hereditary	stress
homeostasis	systemic
hypertension	wellness

KEY POINTS

- Although many definitions of health exist, optimum health includes physical, emotional, mental, social, and spiritual well-being.
- The state of one's health is on a continuum and is dynamic, changing from day to day.
- The concept of high-level wellness relates to the higher level needs in Maslow's hierarchy.
- Lifestyle changes can have a major impact on health and wellness.
- The four most important wellness lifestyle factors are physical activity, healthy diet, maintenance of appropriate weight, and not smoking.
- Some stress is beneficial, whereas too much stress can lead to physical and emotional disorders.
- Keys to changing behavior include health promotion, education, and community health awareness.

- Infant mortality remains a health concern in the United States.
- Accidents are the major cause of death and disability in young children.
- Accidents continue to be a major health concern for adolescents and young adults, along with homicide and suicide.
- Heart disease and cancer are the top causes of death in adults.
- The etiology of diseases and disorders may be organic, functional hereditary, congenital, infectious, deficiency-related, metabolic, neoplastic, traumatic, or related to an occupation.

■ Teaching–Learning Strategies

CLASSROOM

1. Ask the students to define the following abbreviations:

CHD	LDL
COPD	MVA
HDL	STD
HIV	WHO

   Write the students' responses on the chalkboard or on an overhead transparency.

2. Before the class, ask students to keep a journal of their diet and exercise patterns for a 3-day period. Ask students to share their journals with a partner during the class. Ask each student to evaluate the other student's diet and exercise patterns. Have the students share their evaluations with the larger group.

3. Before the class, ask students to visit a healthcare facility, clinic, or physician's office and determine if written or other materials are available to clients related to health education. Bring to class some pamphlets or booklets related to health factors. Ask students to share their findings with the class.

4. Ask a nurse who assists clients with stress management to visit the class and make a presentation about stress management. After the presentation, open the class for questions and discussion. Ask students to share how they cope with life's stressors.

5. On an overhead transparency or the chalkboard, list age groups from infancy to older adults. During the class, ask students to identify health concerns of various age groups. Write the students' responses on the transparency or chalkboard.

CLINICAL

1. Take a small group of students to a clinic or an in-patient setting that cares for clients experiencing stress-related disorders. Ask the students to interview a nurse employed in the setting and discuss the types of clients and nursing care. Ask students to share their findings during clinical conference.

2. Take a small group of students to a shelter that cares for victims of abuse. Ask one of the staff members to discuss the services provided by the shelter. Ask students to share their findings with the larger group.

3. Assign students to attend one self-help group meeting (e.g., Weight Watchers). Ask students to record their observations and share them with the larger group.

4. Ask each student to select one age group and design a teaching plan or a poster that would address the typical healthcare concerns for that age group. Ask the students to share their plans or posters with the larger group.

SUGGESTED RESOURCES

National Center for Injury Prevention and Control, E-mail: *DVPINFO@cdc.gov*; telephone: 770-488-4646

U.S. Department of Health and Human Services, website: *www.hhs.gov*

CHAPTER 7

Community Health

LEARNING OBJECTIVES

1. Define the term *community*. State the relationship of community to that of the health of a community. Identify at least four types of communities.

2. Identify the health-related functions of the World Health Organization (WHO) and UNICEF.

3. State at least six achievements attributed to improvements in public health that resulted in an increase of lifespan in the 20th century.

4. Define and differentiate between the United States Public Health Service (USPHS), the United States Department of Health and Human Services (USDHHS), and the Office of Public Health and Science (OPHS).

5. Discuss at least six functions of USDHHS.

6. Identify at least four functions of the Centers for Disease Control (CDC).

7. Identify at least four functions of the Food and Drug Administration (FDA).

8. Discuss the purpose of the National Institutes of Health (NIH) and state the role of the National Institute for Nursing Research (NINR).

9. Identify at least four functions of Occupational Safety and Health Administration (OSHA).

10. Identify at least three functions of the Social Security Agency.

11. Identify the role and at least two functions of each of the following organizations: American Public Health Association (APHA), National Safety Council, the Red Cross, and the Visiting Nurses' Association (VNA).

12. Differentiate between organizations that are related to specific disorders and organizations promoting specific health goals.

13. Identify at least seven programs that are common to state healthcare services.

14. Discuss the functions of primary care and a community health center.

15. Identify at least three causes of each of the following types of pollution: air, water, land, and noise.

16. Discuss the significance of plumbism, radiation, and biohazardous waste pollution.

NEW TERMINOLOGY

biohazardous	pollution
bionomics	primary healthcare
community	radiation
community health	radon
demography	target population
ecology	worker's compensation
plumbism	

KEY POINTS

- You are a member of many communities and should serve as an advocate and educator to protect those communities.
- Healthcare services are provided on the international, national, state, and local levels.
- Federal agencies include the United States Public Health Service and the Department of Health and Human Services. They have many branches and numerous programs.
- The Blood-Borne Pathogen Standard established by OSHA has significantly affected nursing procedures and delivery of services in healthcare facilities.
- The Social Security Administration supervises the Medicare and Medicaid programs.
- Voluntary health agencies may be set up to provide direct service, education, or fund raising to combat a particular disease or for specific health concerns.
- Public and private agencies often work together to provide healthcare services.
- Many primary healthcare services are provided at community health centers. These services include examinations, health screening, immunizations, education, support groups, and illness care.
- Community health is concerned with environmental issues, including air, water, land, and noise pollution; plumbism; radiation; and biohazardous waste disposal.

■ Teaching–Learning Strategies

CLASSROOM

1. Ask the students to define the following abbreviations:

ACS	HRA
ADAMHA	HAS
ATF	MCHB
BOH	MUA
CDC	NIH
DOA	OMH
DOH	OTC (drugs)
FDA	TTY

   Write the students' responses on the chalkboard or on an overhead transparency.

2. Before class, ask students to visit the library and review an article from a journal related to community or public health. Ask the students to summarize the article and share their findings with the class.

CHAPTER 8

Transcultural Healthcare

LEARNING OBJECTIVES

1. Define and state the components of culture, subculture, race, minorities, and ethnicity.

2. Identify the four major subcultural groups of your community, your state, and the United States.

3. Define and give examples of prejudice, ethnocentrism, and stereotyping.

4. Identify three barriers to providing culturally competent nursing care.

5. List at least eight nursing considerations that should be part of a cultural assessment.

6. Discuss at least two ways in which each of the following influence nursing care: values and beliefs, taboos and rituals, concepts of health and illness, language and communication, diet and nutrition, elimination, and death and dying.

7. Assess the importance of religious and spiritual beliefs for clients experiencing illness.

8. Compare and contrast the following belief systems: magicoreligious, scientific-biomedical, holistic, and Yin–Yang.

9. Discuss the common philosophies of mental illness in at least three different cultures and state how these ideas affect nursing care.

10. Identify at least three important qualifications for an interpreter.

11. Discuss at least three cultural aspects of personal space, touching, eye contact, diet, elimination, and concepts of death and dying. Relate these aspects to concepts of nursing care.

NEW TERMINOLOGY

beliefs	ethnicity
cultural diversity	ethnonursing
cultural sensitivity	karma
culture	minority
curandero	nirvana
ethnocentrism	norms

prejudice	subculture
race	taboos
rituals	transcultural nursing
shaman	values
stereotype	Yin–Yang

KEY POINTS

- Many definitions are given for "culture." Culture refers to a shared set of beliefs and values among a specific group of people.
- Subculture, minorities, and ethnic and racial mixes are components of cultural heritage.
- The mix of ethnic groups in the United States changes continually.
- Prejudice, ethnocentrism, and stereotyping interfere with providing culturally competent nursing care.
- Many ethnic/cultural factors affect the delivery and acceptance of traditional Western healthcare.
- Many cultures subscribe to beliefs such as karma, Yin–Yang, spirits, or fate as causes of and cures for illness.
- Cultural and religious traditions are not always followed by every member of a group.
- To facilitate communication and good nursing care, the nurse should be acquainted with the predominant cultural and religious groups within the community.
- The nurse may suggest a visit from a spiritual leader but should not call one without first asking the client.
- Transcultural nursing is nursing that considers the religious and sociocultural backgrounds of all clients.

■ Teaching–Learning Strategies

CLASSROOM

1. Ask students to define the following abbreviations:

   LDS (Latter Day Saints, Mormon)
   RC (Roman Catholic)

Write the students' responses on the chalkboard or on an overhead transparency.

2. Ask students to share their own cultural/religious/spiritual customs and rituals. List these on the chalkboard or overhead transparency. Ask students to identify how these beliefs may influence their provision of nursing care to clients of different cultures/beliefs.

3. Provide students with a definition of culture and ethnicity. Ask students how they would change or modify these definitions. Write these changes on the chalkboard or an overhead transparency.

4. Ask a nurse who is from a minority ethnic group to visit the class and discuss his or her cultural practices. After the presentation, open the class for discussion.

5. Ask students to identify barriers to culturally competent care and how nurses (and student nurses) can overcome these barriers.

6. On an overhead transparency or the chalkboard, list the four major health belief systems. Ask students to explain what each belief system represents.

CLINICAL

1. Assign students to interview an individual whose cultural beliefs may be different from their own. Ask students to share their findings during clinical conference.

2. Assign students to a clinical setting where they will have their clinical experiences. Ask students to interview a nurse on the unit who cares for clients of various cultural groups. Ask students to share their findings during clinical conference.

3. Ask an individual who serves as an interpreter for the clinical institution to visit the group and discuss the role of the interpreter in a healthcare

setting. After the presentation, open the clinical conference for discussion.

SUGGESTED RESOURCES

Communicating with clients from different cultures. (1995). [Videotape, 20 minutes]. (Available from Insight Media, P.O. Box 621, New York, NY 10024-0621)

Cultural diversity: Appreciating differences. (1996). [Videotape, 25 minutes]. (Available from Insight Media, P.O. Box 621, New York, NY 10024-0621)

Cultural diversity in health care. (1994). [Videotape, 25 minutes]. (Available from Insight Media, P.O. Box 621, New York, NY 10024-0621)

I'm normal, you're weird: Understanding other cultures. (1997). [Videotape, 23 minutes]. (Available from Insight Media, P.O. Box 621, New York, NY 10024-0621)

Mental health assessment in the home. (1996). *Assessing older adults in the home.* [Videotape]. (Available from Lippincott Williams & Wilkins, 530 Walnut Street, Philadelphia, PA 19106)

Open doors: Public health nursing in its 100th year. [Videotape, 33 minutes]. (Available from Fanlight Productions, 47 Halifax Street, Boston, MA 02130)

Pain management in the home. (1996). *Assessing older adults in the home.* [Videotape]. (Available from Lippincott Williams & Wilkins, 530 Walnut Street, Philadelphia, PA 19106)

Valuing diversity: Multicultural communication. (1994). [Videotape, 19 minutes]. (Available from Insight Media, P.O. Box 621, New York, NY 10024-0621)

What is home care? (1996). [Videotape, 22 minutes]. (Available from Lippincott Williams & Wilkins, 530 Walnut Street, Philadelphia, PA 19106). Clinical Issues in Home Health Nursing [Set of 3 Videotapes].

ADDITIONAL RESOURCES

American Indian Students United for Nursing (ASUN) Project, website: *www.asu.edu/nursing/asun.html*

National Association of Hispanic Nurses, website: *www.thehispanicnurses.org*

National Black Nurses Association Inc., website: *www.nbna.org*

Office of Minority Health, telephone: 800-444-6472; TDD, 301-230-7199

Transcultural Nursing Society, website: *www.tcns.org*

U.S. Department of Health and Human Services, website: *www.hhs.gov, www.omhrc.gov*

U.S. Public Health Service, telephone: 301-587-9704, 800-444-6472

CHAPTER 9

The Family

LEARNING OBJECTIVES

1. Identify the five universal characteristics of families.

2. Discuss the importance of the parent-child and sibling relationships.

3. List the functions and tasks of families.

4. Describe various types of family structure.

5. Explain the influences of culture, ethnicity, and religion on the family.

6. Discuss the stages of the family life cycle and important milestones and tasks of these stages.

7. Identify common stressors on today's family.

8. Differentiate between effective and ineffective family coping patterns.

NEW TERMINOLOGY

binuclear family	functional family
cohabitation	gay or lesbian family
communal family	nuclear dyad
commuter family	nuclear family
dual-career/dual-worker family	reconstituted family
dysfunctional family	siblings
extended family	single adult household
family	single-parent family
foster family	

KEY POINTS

- The family is the basic unit of society, but it is a complex unit.
- All nursing care should involve clients and their families.
- Although each family is unique, families share five universal characteristics: every family is a small social system; has certain basic functions; has a structure; has its own cultural values and rules; moves through stages in its life cycle.

- Roles and relationships within a family are many and varied; the primary ones include parent-child and sibling relationships.
- The functions and tasks of the family help individuals to meet their basic human needs.
- Although many different family structures exist, all can be efficient, supportive, and satisfying.
- Cultural, ethnic, and religious factors influence family outcomes.
- Family development progresses through predictable stages with important developmental tasks.
- The family that can cope with stress is functional; families that cannot cope are dysfunctional or at risk.

■Teaching–Learning Strategies

CLASSROOM

1. During the class, ask the students to list five characteristics of families. Ask students to share how these five characteristics apply to their own families.

2. List the seven family tasks that relate to basic human needs. Ask students to relate how these tasks are accomplished in their own families.

3. Conduct a discussion with the class about various types of family structures. Ask students to identify ways in which a family structure can have an influence on healthcare for the family members.

4. On an overhead transparency or the chalkboard, outline the seven stages of the family life cycle. Ask the students to identify the various tasks for each stage and list the student responses.

5. Ask students to identify various stressors that occur in families (e.g., divorce) and how these stressors can affect the care of the family members. Discuss effective family coping strategies.

CLINICAL

1. Assign students in the clinical setting to interview a client from a culture or religion different from that of the student's. Ask students to discuss the client's family. Ask students to share their findings during clinical conference.

2. Ask a nurse who cares for families during crisis (e.g., crisis center, woman's shelter) to visit the clinical conference and discuss the role of the nurse. Following the presentation, open the clinical conference for discussion.

3. Assign students in pairs to various agencies (e.g., women's shelter, Red Cross) that care for various types of families and interview nurses in the agency. Ask students to share their findings with the larger class group.

CHAPTER 10

Infancy and Childhood

LEARNING OBJECTIVES

1. List the characteristics and sequence of human growth and development.

2. Explain developmental regression.

3. Discuss Havighurst's theory of developmental tasks.

4. Describe Erikson's stages of psychosocial development, including the challenges and virtues of each stage.

5. Explain the four stages of human cognitive development as described by Piaget.

6. Describe the role of play in childhood development.

7. Discuss the importance of anticipatory guidance for caregivers as their children grow and progress to new developmental stages.

8. Discuss growth and development for infants, toddlers, preschoolers, and school-age children, highlighting key areas of concern.

NEW TERMINOLOGY

bonding
cephalocaudal
cognitive
development
environment
enuresis
growth
hereditary
infancy

interdependent
masturbation
newborn
object permanence
proximodistal
regression
stranger anxiety
toddler

KEY POINTS

- Growth and development is an ongoing process throughout childhood.
- Growth and development progresses in a particular sequence (cephalocaudal: head to toe; and proximodistal: center outward).
- Theorists including Havighurst, Erikson, and Piaget have identified specific tasks to accomplish and

stages to pass through to become a mature, fully functional person.

- Play is an important element of growth and development that helps prepare children for more levels of functioning.
- Nurses and other healthcare providers can give anticipatory guidance to help prepare family caregivers for the normal areas of concern that arise during each developmental stage.
- Infancy, which ends at age 1 year, is the period of fastest growth and development during the entire lifespan.
- Toddlerhood (1–3 years) is a time marked by exploration, growing independence, and conflicting emotions.
- During the preschool years (3–6 years), children exhibit imagination, improved communication skills, and curiosity.
- School greatly influences children aged 6 to 10 years, as they branch away from the family home. They develop relationships with peers, participate in school and community activities, and learn more about the world around them.

■ Teaching–Learning Strategies

CLASSROOM

1. Show the videotape *Child Development: The First Two Years* (47 minutes; available from Lippincott Williams & Wilkins, 530 Walnut Street, Philadelphia, PA 19106; ISBN 0-7817-1247-5). After the presentation, ask students to highlight the major milestones of growth and development during the first 2 years of life. Ask students to identify major health concerns for this age group.

2. Show the series of videotapes *The Growing Child: Infancy Through Adolescence* (series of six videotapes, 30 minutes each; available from Lippincott Williams & Wilkins, 530 Walnut Street, Philadelphia, PA 19106; ISBN 0-397-5587705). Discuss the various milestones of

growth and development for each age group. Ask the students to identify major health concerns for each age group.

3. On an overhead transparency or the chalkboard, list the three theorists from the textbook: Havighurst, Erikson, and Piaget. Ask students to compare and contrast each theorist and write the student's responses.

4. On an overhead transparency, list the age groups: infancy, toddler, preschool, and school-age. Ask the students to identify anticipatory guidance needs for caregivers for each age group.

CLINICAL

1. Assign students in pairs to visit various local daycare centers or preschools. Assign each pair of students to observe various age groups. Ask the students to share their findings during clinical conference.

2. Visit an inpatient or outpatient pediatric unit in a hospital setting. Ask the students to observe the children who are hospitalized or who are receiving outpatient care. Ask students to share their observations during clinical conference.

3. Assign a small group of students to spend 2 to 3 hours with a school nurse in an elementary school. Ask the students to interview and observe the nurse caring for the children. Ask the students to share their observations in clinical conference.

4. Arrange for a tour of a play area of a pediatric hospital unit. Ask students to observe the children and relate their observations during clinical conference. Ask students to evaluate the play area and determine how they would change or improve the area if they were able to do so.

5. If there is a Ronald McDonald house in the area, arrange for a small group of students to visit the facility. Ask students to interview the family members at the house and share their findings during clinical conference.

CHAPTER 11

Adolescence

LEARNING OBJECTIVES

1. Explain the term *puberty* and its relationship to adolescence.

2. Relate the theories of Havighurst, Erikson, and Piaget to adolescent growth and development.

3. Explain how skill development contributes to expanding cognition and decision-making.

4. Discuss the different stages of adolescence.

5. Describe the specific physical changes that occur between the ages of 11 and 20 years.

6. Discuss sexual development for boys and girls.

7. Identify the importance of relationships for adolescents.

8. Describe the cognitive, emotional, and moral development that occurs during adolescence.

9. Discuss appropriate discipline strategies for adolescents.

10. Design a plan for presenting information concerning human sexuality to adolescents.

NEW TERMINOLOGY

adolescence
menarche
nocturnal emission
peer group
preadolescence
puberty

KEY POINTS

- Adolescence is a turbulent time, marked by rapid physical growth and frequent emotional upheavals.
- Puberty is the time when a person matures sexually and becomes able to reproduce.
- The developmental tasks of adolescence involve the formation of a self-image, establishment of goals for the future, and building relationships with others.

- Skill development in adolescence helps teenagers to learn more and may influence future career and educational choices.
- Great variation exists in physical and emotional maturity among young people.
- Relationships with family and friends and dating contribute to the adolescent's self-perceptions and interpersonal skills.
- Solid family communication and relations help adolescents get through difficult challenges.
- Age-appropriate discipline is important for adolescents trying to withstand peer pressure.
- Sex education from trusted adults helps teenagers avoid mistakes based on misinformation.

■ Teaching–Learning Strategies

CLASSROOM

1. Before class, on an overhead transparency, write the three theorists: Havighurst, Erikson, and Piaget. In class, ask students to list the developmental, psychosocial, and cognitive tasks of an adolescent. Write the students' responses on the transparency.

2. On the chalkboard or on an overhead transparency, compare and contrast the physical and sexual developmental of adolescent boys and girls.

3. List the three phases of adolescence: early, middle, and late adolescence. Ask students to identify the cognitive, emotional, and moral developmental tasks for each phase.

4. Ask students to identify various health concerns for the adolescent (e.g., poor eating habits). Ask students how nurses can assist adolescents with their concerns. Write the students' responses on the chalkboard or on an overhead transparency.

5. Show the videotape *Teen Suicide* (35 minutes; available from Films for the Humanities and

Sciences, P.O. Box 2053, Princeton, NJ 08543-2053). After the videotape presentation, open the class for discussion.

6. Ask a nurse who cares for pregnant adolescents to visit the class and discuss the support services available to adolescents. After the presentation, open the class for questions and answers from the students.

7. Show the videotape "Adolescence" from the *Growing Child Series* (30 minutes; available from Lippincott Williams & Wilkins, 530 Walnut Street, Philadelphia, PA 19106; ISBN 0-397-48059-8). After the videotape presentation, open the class for discussion and comments.

CLINICAL

1. Take a small group of students to a clinic that primarily cares for adolescents. Ask each student to observe the role of the nurse in caring for adolescent clients. Ask students to share their observations with the larger group.

2. Ask students to interview one or two adolescents about their health concerns. Ask students to submit a brief written report on their findings and share their findings with the larger group.

3. Assign a small group of students to an inpatient setting with adolescent clients. Ask each student to interview the client and review the client's record or chart to determine the reason for the hospitalization and the plan of care. Ask students to share their observations during clinical conference.

4. Assign students in pairs to visit a local junior or senior high school. Ask students to interview the school nurse about the health care needs of adolescent students. Ask the students to share their findings with the larger group.

CHAPTER 12

Early and Middle Adulthood

LEARNING OBJECTIVES

1. List Havighurst's eight developmental tasks for early and middle adulthood.

2. Describe Erikson's theory of psychosocial development as it applies to young and middle adults.

3. Compare Levinson's "individual structure" theory with the theories of Havighurst and Erikson.

4. Explain Gail Sheehy's theory of the "phases of adulthood."

5. Discuss the implications of life choices made during early adulthood.

6. Examine one aspect of life (e.g., vocation, intimate relationships) and apply it across middle adulthood.

NEW TERMINOLOGY

generativity
intimacy
isolation
midlife transition

KEY POINTS

- Adults must meet certain developmental tasks to mature comfortably.
- Development continues throughout life and during adulthood; periods of stability alternate with periods of transition.
- Because many adults choose to live with other people, integrating individual goals into joint goals often is helpful.

■ Teaching–Learning Strategies

CLASSROOM

1. Before class, ask students to interview early and middle-age adults, either from their own family or from other families. Ask students to focus on growth and developmental patterns of these adults. Ask students to share their findings with the larger class.

2. Before class, on an overhead transparency, list the four theorists from the chapter: Havighurst, Erikson, Levinson, and Sheehy. Ask the students during class to identify each theorist's development tasks of adults. Write the students' responses on the transparency.

3. On an overhead transparency or the chalkboard, list the two phases of adulthood: early and middle. Divide the class into two groups and ask students to form pairs. Ask each pair of students to identify the major developmental tasks for either early adulthood or middle adulthood. Ask the students to share their results with the larger group.

4. Ask one or two nurses who have been in practice for at least 20 years to visit the class and discuss how their nursing care and roles have changed over the years. After the presentation, open the class for discussion.

CLINICAL

1. Take a group of students to a clinical setting that cares primarily for adult clients. Ask the students to interview a client about his or her hospitalization experience and nursing care. After the interviews, ask the students to share their findings during clinical conference.

2. Assign pairs of students to visit community clinics for adult clients, a battered women's shelter, or a center that serves the homeless. Ask the students to interview one staff member and one client about the services provided. Ask the students to share their observations with the larger group.

3. Ask students to attend a PTA meeting or visit other organizations appropriate for early and middle adults. Ask students to report their observations to the larger group.

CHAPTER 13

Older Adulthood and Aging

LEARNING OBJECTIVES

1. Describe Havighurst's developmental tasks related to older adulthood.

2. Explain the psychosocial development of older adults as defined by Erikson.

3. Discuss Levinson's and Sheehy's perspectives on older adulthood.

4. Identify positive factors in the development of the aging person.

5. List stressors for older adults.

6. Identify implications for society related to the increasing numbers of older adults.

7. Explain at least five challenges for future healthcare related to changing demographics.

NEW TERMINOLOGY

ageism
gerontology
mortality

KEY POINTS

- The process of aging is a continuation of earlier development. Each person differs in the speed with which he or she ages, in adaptations made to aging, and in coping mechanisms.
- Ageism refers to discrimination against individuals as they grow older.
- Older people want to remain independent, maintain their self-esteem, find outlets for their energies and interests, develop a happy lifestyle within their financial means, continue positive relationships with others, meet all basic human needs, and confront their mortality.
- Stress, loss, and poverty are significant concerns for older adults.
- Population trends are necessitating more research for adult development past the age of 85 years.
- Society must examine healthcare concerns related to the expanding older population.

■ Teaching–Learning Strategies

CLASSROOM

1. Before class, use an overhead transparency to write the four theorists from the chapter: Havighurst, Erikson, Levinson, and Sheehy. During the class, ask the students to divide into four groups. Assign each group one of the theorists. Ask students to identify the developmental tasks of the theorist that they are assigned. Ask the students to share their responses with the larger group.

2. Before class, ask students to interview an adult age 65 years or older. Ask the students to interview the adult on the person's views and concerns related to health, healthcare, finances, stress, spirituality, and mortality. Ask the students to share their interviews with the larger class.

3. Ask a representative from a senior citizen center to speak to the class about the services and activities offered by the center. After the presentation, open the class for discussion and questions and answers.

4. Ask a retired nurse to visit the class and describe how nursing and nursing roles changed during her career. After the presentation, open the class for discussion and questions and answers.

5. Show the videotape *I'm Pretty Old* (1992; 20 minutes; available from Aquarius Health Care Videos, P.O. Box 1159, Sherborn, MA 01770; 508-651-2963). After the videotape presentation, open the class for discussion.

6. Show the videotape *Alzheimer's Disease* (1997; 28 minutes; Aquarius Health Care Videos, P.O. Box 1159, Sherborn, MA 01770; 508-651-2963). After the videotape presentation, open the class for discussion.

CLINICAL

1. Assign students in pairs to visit a long-term care facility for older adults. Ask the students to interview one staff member and one resident about the nursing care required for older adults. Ask the students to share their findings and observations during clinical conference.

2. Assign a small group of students to an inpatient facility that cares for older adults. Ask the students to interview one older adult client and focus on their reason for hospitalization and nursing care. Ask students to share their findings with the larger group.

3. Assign a small group of students to make the daily rounds with a volunteer who delivers meals to older adults in their homes. Ask the students to share their observations with the larger class.

4. Before the clinical or laboratory experience, ask students to visit the library and locate any article from a newspaper or magazine related to older adults. Ask students to summarize the article and present the article during clinical conference. Ask students to share their thoughts about how changing demographics might affect their nursing roles or personal lives in the future.

CHAPTER 14

Death and Dying

LEARNING OBJECTIVES

1. Explain death's relationship to the process of growth and development.

2. Discuss how culture, ethnicity, and religion influence attitudes toward death.

3. Describe the ways in which spirituality can help individuals cope with death.

4. Define what is meant by "terminal illness."

5. Identify the six stages of coping with impending death.

6. Differentiate between preparatory and reactive depression.

7. Explain ways in which the death of an individual affects the family unit and how families grieve.

NEW TERMINOLOGY

detachment
preparatory depression
reactive depression
terminal illness

KEY POINTS

- Death is a normal part of the total life process.
- Culture, ethnicity, and religion influence attitudes toward death and the way people express grief and loss.
- Spirituality is an outlet that helps individuals to handle death and dying.
- Most people, if they do not die suddenly, pass through definite stages during the dying process. The ultimate goal is acceptance.
- Families who face the impending death of a member may endure enormous stress. They need encouragement to express their emotions.

■ Teaching–Learning Strategies

CLASSROOM

1. Show the videotape *Death* (23 minutes; available from Films for the Humanities and Sciences, P.O. Box 2053, Princeton, NJ 08543-2053; 800-257-5126). After the videotape presentation, ask students to share their experiences regarding the death of family members or other individuals.

2. Invite a mortician to visit the class and discuss bereavement and how to help family members cope with the loss. After the presentation, open the class for questions and discussion.

3. Before class, on an overhead transparency, list various religions in one column. During the class, on an overhead transparency, ask students to identify the various religious practices when death occurs.

4. Before class, on an overhead transparency, list the five stages of dying as identified by Kübler-Ross. Ask the students during the class to identify nursing responses to help the client and family members cope with death.

CLINICAL

1. Assign students in the clinical setting to a client who is culturally or religiously different from the students. Ask the students to interview the client about beliefs related to death. Ask students to share their observations during clinical conference.

2. Arrange for students to visit the morgue of the hospital. After this experience, ask students to share their feelings during clinical conference.

3. Ask students to interview a nurse who has cared for a client who has died. Ask students to share their interviews with the larger group.

SUGGESTED RESOURCES: VIDEOTAPES

The aging mind. (1998). [28 minutes]. (Available from Aquarius Health Care Videos, P.O. Box 1159, Sherborn, MA 01770; 508-651-2963)

BSE for teens. (1993). [10 minutes]. (Available from Lippincott Williams & Wilkins, 530 Walnut Street, Philadelphia, PA 19106)

Child abuse. (1985). [28 minutes]. (Available from Lippincott Williams & Wilkins, 530 Walnut Street, Philadelphia, PA 19106)

Discussing advance directives. (1994). [25 minutes]. (Available from Aquarius Productions, P.O. Box 1159, Sherborn, MA 01770; 508-651-2963)

Going it alone: Preparing for single parenthood. [35 minutes]. (Available from Films for the Humanities and Sciences, P.O. Box 2053, Princeton, NJ 08543-2053; 800-257-5126)

Living fully until death. (1996). [28 minutes]. (Available from Aquarius Productions, P.O. Box 1159, Sherborn, MA 01770; 508-651-2963)

No safe place: The origins of violence against women. (1996). [56 minutes]. (Available from Nimco, Inc., P.O. Box 9, 102 Highway 81 North, Calhoun, KY 42327; 800-962-6662 [NIM-60-1-V7])

Stroke: Today's preventable disease. (1994). [11 minutes]. (Available from Nimco, Inc., P.O. Box, 102 Highway 81 North, Calhoun, KY 42327; 800-962-6662 [NIM-42-2-V7])

Teenage pregnancy. [26 minutes]. (Available from Films for the Humanities and Sciences, P.O. Box 2053, Princeton, NJ 08543-2053; 800-257-5126)

The way we die. [25 minutes]. (Available from Fanlight Productions, 47 Halifax Street, Boston, MA 02130)

Organization of the Human Body

LEARNING OBJECTIVES

1. Define and differentiate between anatomy, physiology, and pathophysiology.

2. Using the information in Chapter 15 and the appendix, define the following terms: intravenous, hepatitis, dysphagia.

3. Differentiate between the sagittal, transverse, and frontal planes.

4. Define the different directional terms and give an example of each.

5. Define homeostasis.

6. Describe the basic organization of atoms, elements, compounds, and mixtures.

7. Explain the difference between a physical and a chemical change.

8. Describe the organization of the human body in terms of cells, tissues, organs, and systems.

9. Explain the basic organization of the cell.

10. Discuss the activities of each cell part. Differentiate between RNA and DNA.

11. Differentiate between mitosis and meiosis.

12. List the four major types of tissue and give an example of each.

13. Explain how organs and systems function in the body.

NEW TERMINOLOGY

anatomic position	cytoplasm
anatomy	diaphragm
atom	dorsal
body cavity	element
cell	enzyme
cell membrane	frontal
chemical change	gene
chromosome	homeostasis
cilia	medical terminology
compound	meiosis

metabolism	plasma membrane
mitosis	protoplasm
mixture	quadrant
nucleus	sagittal
organ	system
pathophysiology	tissue
physical change	transverse
physiology	ventral
plane	

KEY POINTS

- The human body is made up of solids, liquids, and gases that function independently but are interrelated.
- The study of the human body can be subdivided into the study of anatomy (structure), physiology (function), and pathophysiology (disorders of function).
- Medicine has developed a sophisticated system of describing anatomy and physiology called *medical terminology*. To assist the learner, much of this terminology can be broken down into prefixes, suffixes, and root words.
- The body is described in terms of superior, inferior, dorsal, and ventral directions. It also is described in terms of transverse, frontal, and sagittal planes and specific cavities containing viscera.
- Homeostasis is the dynamic balance of an individual's physical and mental functioning.
- Substances are capable of undergoing physical changes in outward appearance or chemical changes with the transfer of energy.
- The body can be described in terms of a single cell, which collaborates with similar cells in groups called tissues. Similar tissues, functioning as a group, comprise organs. Groups of organs make up body systems.
- Each cell is composed of many complex structures. Each structure has a specific duty that relates to the body as a whole. Cells have similar abilities but have developed specialized functions. Some special abilities include metabolism, contractility, conductivity, and irritability.

- Genes, the controller of heredity, are found on chromosomes. Body cells replicate (reproduce) through mitosis. Sex cells (eggs and sperm) replicate through meiosis. Human cells have 46 chromosomes.
- The body is made up of four basic kinds of tissue: epithelial, connective, muscle, and nerve.
- The body is organized according to systems, or groups of organs, that work together to perform certain functions that contribute to the overall workings of the body.

■ Teaching–Learning Strategies

CLASSROOM

1. Assign pairs of students several prefixes, roots, suffixes, and chemical symbols. Ask the students to define these terms or symbols and write their responses on the chalkboard or on an overhead transparency.

2. Ask the students to define the following abbreviations and terms:

DNA	RUQ
H_2O	WBC
LLQ	atom
LUQ	epithelial
MASH	integumentary
RBC	nucleus

Write the students' responses on the chalkboard or on an overhead transparency.

3. Labeling exercises: Ask the students to label the:

a. Body planes and directions
b. Hydrogen and oxygen atom
c. Typical body cell
d. Types of epithelial tissue
e. Major internal organs
f. Quadrants of the body

CLINICAL

1. While in a clinical setting, ask the students to review client records for their medical and nursing diagnoses. Ask the students to review the records for medical terminology, anatomy, and physiology. Ask the students to share their findings with the larger group after the students have defined these terms.

2. In the learning laboratory, review medical terminology. Ask the students to separate into pairs and identify structural organization of the body's systems on each other.

3. In the learning laboratory, show the videotape *The Cell* (28 minutes; Nimco, Inc., P.O. Box 9, 102 Highway 81 North, Calhoun, KY 42327). Using charts or models, allow the students to practice identifying major body systems.

ADDITIONAL RESOURCES

The Cells Alive link from the Biology School Page has information on animal cells, mitosis, antibody production, and specific cell functions under the "cell gallery" link: *www.cellsalive.com/*.

The Digital Anatomist, E-mail, *DIGITAL_ANATOMIST@BIOSTR.WASHINGTON.EDU*

CHAPTER 16

The Integumentary System

LEARNING OBJECTIVES

1. Describe the structure and main functions of the skin.

2. Describe the function of keratin and melanin.

3. Identify the structures of a nail.

4. Contrast the different functions of the sudoriferous glands and sebaceous glands.

5. Define convection, evaporation, conduction, and radiation and give an example of each.

6. Explain the purpose of "goose bumps" or "goose flesh."

7. Discuss the skin's role in sensory awareness.

8. Name five changes that occur to aging skin.

NEW TERMINOLOGY

alopecia	hypodermis
carotene	integument
cerumen	keratin
ceruminal glands	melanin
collagen	radiation
conduction	sebaceous glands
convection	sebum
corium	skin turgor
dermis	squamous
desquamation	subcutaneous tissue
diaphoresis	sudoriferous glands
epidermis	thermoregulation
evaporation	transdermally
freckles	vitiligo

KEY POINTS

- The skin and its accessory structures (hair, nails, and glands) make up the integumentary system.
- Primary functions of the integumentary system consist of protection, thermoregulation, metabolism, sensation, and communication.
- The skin, the largest organ in the body, is vital for survival. Principle layers of the skin are the superficial epidermis and the deep dermis. The subcutaneous tissue lies below the dermis and binds the skin to underlying muscle tissue.
- The epidermis contains keratin, which protects the body from excessive water loss or gain, and melanin, which protects the body from ultraviolet rays. The epidermis is the outermost protective layer.
- The dermis underlies the epidermis and contains nerves, hair follicles, blood and lymph vessels, and glands. It is composed of tough connective tissue containing collagen, which contributes to the skin's elasticity.
- The subcutaneous tissue, or hypodermis, is made of fat cells that insulate and protect underlying tissues.
- Skin color is due to melanin, carotene, and hemoglobin.
- Glands are unicellular or multicellular structures of epithelial tissue that produce secretions and contribute to the protection and thermoregulation functions of the integumentary system.
- The skin regulates and balances the body's temperature via convection, evaporation, conduction, shivering, and radiation. Infants and the elderly have a higher risk of heat loss than do other adults.
- Through sensory awareness the skin provides a dynamic interaction between the external and internal environments.
- Effects of aging include wrinkling, loss of subcutaneous fat, atrophy of glands, and decreased numbers of protective cells. Thus, skin problems are more common for older adults.
- To protect the skin, one should eat a healthy diet and drink an adequate amount of fluid daily. Additional protection when in the sun includes wearing long sleeved clothing, staying in the shade, and applying sunscreen.

▪ Teaching–Learning Strategies

CLASSROOM

1. Ask the students to define the following terms and abbreviations:

UV	convection
CSF	sebaceous
ECF	sebum
HCl	ceruminal
ICF	collagen
KCl	desquamation
mEq	squamous
mL	vitiligo
NaCl	hypodermis
vitamin D	freckles
alopecia	mammary
carotene	melanin
diaphoresis	sudoriferous
evaporation	thermoregulation
radiation	

2. Labeling exercises: Ask the students to label the

   a. Cross section of skin structures

   b. Processes of heat loss

3. Review the effects of aging on the integumentary system with the class. Ask the students to share their personal experiences of observations of older family members and changes in their integumentary system as a result of aging.

CLINICAL

1. Review the integumentary system structures with a model, chart, or transparency. Demonstrate the four processes of heat loss (convection, conduction, radiation, and evaporation).

2. Assign students to perform an assessment of the integumentary system on an infant or child, a young adult, and an older adult. Ask the students to write their findings in a one- to two-page paper. Ask the students to share their findings with the larger group.

3. Assign students to locate an article on the integumentary system through use of the library or Internet. Ask the students to summarize the article in a one- to two-page paper. Ask the students to share their findings with the larger group.

4. In the clinical setting, assign students to one client and ask the students to perform an assessment of the clients' integumentary system. Ask the students to summarize their findings in writing and share their findings with the larger group. This may be on a separate piece of paper or in the client's record (chart).

5. In the clinical setting, ask students to write the physician's orders for a specific client. Ask the students to share these orders with the larger group.

ADDITIONAL RESOURCES

American Cancer Society, website: *www.cancer.org*
Aging Skin Net (link from Skin Care Physicians), website: *www.skincarephysicians.com/agingskinnet/index.html*
Human Anatomy Online, website: *www.innerbody.com*
A map of skin, including epidermis, dermis, and subcutaneous tissue is available at *www.medic.mieu.ac.jp/derma/anatomy.html*
Skin Care Physicians, website: *www.skincarephysicians.com/*

CHAPTER 17

Fluid and Electrolyte Balance

LEARNING OBJECTIVES

1. Define homeostasis. Explain the negative and positive feedback systems.

2. Define the terms *intracellular fluid* and *extracellular fluid*. Define and discuss the components of these two compartments and the respective portion of total body weight that each represents.

3. Describe how the thirst center, atrial natriuretic peptide, and the RAA system help regulate fluid balance.

4. Explain "third-spacing" and describe four ways that edema can occur. State three nursing interventions that would be helpful to teach a client in decreasing or preventing edema.

5. Identify four functions of water.

6. Name the most important cation and anion in intracellular and extracellular fluid.

7. Describe three major electrolytes responsible for maintenance of neuronal and muscular activity. Describe two nursing actions that might be appropriate for maintaining these electrolytes in balance.

8. Differentiate between freely permeable and selectively permeable membranes and discuss factors affecting permeability.

9. Contrast the transportation of fluids by way of diffusion, filtration, osmosis, and active transport.

10. Explain the normal sources water gain by body and mechanisms of water loss in the body. Discuss the "normal" intake and output for an average adult.

11. Describe the bicarbonate buffer system and how it functions to maintain homeostasis. Discuss the significance of arterial blood gas results in caring for your client. What are the nursing implications for a person who has a high carbon dioxide level on the ABG report.

12. Explain why infants, young children, and elderly are at risk for fluid and electrolyte abnormalities.

13. Describe two nursing implications for the elderly in maintaining fluid and electrolyte balance.

NEW TERMINOLOGY

acid	homeostasis
anasarca	hypertonic
anion	hypotonic
ascites	insensible
base	interstitial
buffer	intravascular
cation	ion
dehydration	isotonic
diffusion	osmosis
edema	permeability
electrolyte	salt
feedback	solute
filtration	solvent

KEY POINTS

- Homeostasis is a state of dynamic equilibrium; the body constantly adjusts to external and internal stimuli.
- Feedback is the relaying of information to and from organ systems (especially the nervous and endocrine systems). Feedback keeps the body's functioning capacity within normal boundaries.
- The body has two main fluid compartments: intracellular (within the cells) and extracellular. Extracellular fluid is located in blood vessels (plasma) and in tissues (interstitial fluid).
- Homeostatic mechanisms involved in the regulation of extracellular fluid include the actions of the thirst center, antidiuretic hormone (ADH), rennin-angiotensin-aldosterone system, and atrial natriuretic peptide (ANP).

- Water acts as a solvent and suspension agent. It helps regulate body temperature, pH, and fluid pressures inside and outside the cell. It assists and participates in chemical reactions.
- Electrolytes are substances that in water dissolve into ions. Ions are charged particles that circulate in the body fluids and take part in the body's chemical reactions.
- Normal saline (0.9% NaCl) is an isotonic solution. Stronger solutions are hypertonic; weaker solutions are hypotonic.
- Fluids are transported passively (without ATP energy) or actively (with ATP energy).
- Intake and output must be balanced to avoid fluid deficit (dehydration) or a fluid excess (edema).
- The body has buffer systems that help maintain the serum pH in the narrow range between 7.35 and 7.45 (or 7.37 and 7.43). Acids and bases are important components of this system.
- The body uses the lungs to maintain or excrete carbon dioxide and the kidneys to maintain or excrete bicarbonate as part of the bicarbonate buffer system used to regulate the pH. Arterial blood gases are monitored to determine how well the body's acid–base balance is functioning.
- Minute fluid and electrolyte and acid–base changes occur constantly throughout the body, but the overall status in the healthy person is stability and equilibrium. To be healthy, a person's body must maintain this balance as much as possible.

■ Teaching–Learning Strategies

CLASSROOM

1. Ask the students to define the following terms and abbreviations:

base	intravascular
acid	electrolyte
feedback	cation
ion	hypertonic
isotonic	filtration
buffer	permeability
anion	transcellular
edema	hypotonic
dehydration	salt
solute	homeostasis

Write the students' responses on the chalkboard or on an overhead transparency.

2. Show the videotape(s) *Care of the Patient Receiving IV Therapy* (1994; 24 minutes;

available from Lippincott Williams & Wilkins, 530 Walnut Street, Philadelphia, PA 19106; website: *www.lrpub.com*) or *Assessing Fluids and Electrolytes* (1989; 25 minutes; available from Insight Media, P.O. Box 621, New York, NY 10024). After viewing the videotapes, open the class for questions and discussion.

3. Assign students in pairs to identify the functions of the major electrolytes and normal serum values. Write the students' responses on the chalkboard or on an overhead transparency.

4. Review the process of osmosis and filtration. Open the class for questions and discussion.

CLINICAL

1. In the learning laboratory, demonstrate various types of intravenous equipment for the students. Allow students to practice using intravenous therapy equipment.

2. In the clinical setting, assign students to work with a nurse who is caring for a client receiving intravenous therapy. Ask students to assess the client for potential complications, edema, and dehydration. Ask the students to share their experiences during clinical conference.

3. Assign students to review a client's medical record for fluid and electrolyte status. Ask the students to review the client's laboratory findings and write any deviations on a piece of paper. Ask the students to share their findings during clinical conference. Ask students to write the physician's orders on a separate piece of paper and share these with the larger group.

4. Assign pairs of students to join a nurse who makes home visits to clients receiving intravenous therapy. Ask the students to share their observations and experiences with the larger group.

ADDITIONAL RESOURCES

The Altruis Biomedical Network has a website for fluid and electrolytes with links to kidneys, diuretics, thirst, and acid–base balance: *www.e-kidneys.net/*.

The Merck manual has a website for fluid and electrolyte balance in infants and children with links to fluid deficit, excess, and fluid requirements: *www.merck.com/pubs/ mmanual/section19/sec19.htm*.

CHAPTER 18

The Musculoskeletal System

LEARNING OBJECTIVES

1. List the four classifications of bones according to shape.

2. Locate and name the major bones of the body and their functions.

3. Explain the function of red bone marrow.

4. Name three types of joints and give an example of each.

5. Differentiate between the axial and appendicular skeletons.

6. List the five divisions of the vertebral column and the number of vertebrae in each division.

7. Differentiate between kyphosis, lordosis, and scoliosis.

8. List the skeletal bones and locate them on a skeleton.

9. Differentiate between an adult and an infant skull. Describe two functions of fontanels. Locate the anterior and posterior fontanel on a newborn. Compare and contrast skeletal, smooth, and cardiac muscles and their functions.

10. Locate and name the major muscle groups in the body and indicate the actions of each group.

11. State three factors that influence bone growth.

12. Explain the process by which muscles produce heat. Explain the effects of overusing and underusing muscles.

13. Differentiate between tendons and ligaments.

NEW TERMINOLOGY

acetabulum	carpal
articulation	cartilage
atrophy	clavicle
bursae	coccyx
calcaneus	contractility

diaphysis	medial
elasticity	muscle tone
epiphysis	ossification
extensibility	osteoblast
extension	osteoclast
femur	osteocyte
fibula	patella
flexion	pelvis
gait	periosteum
hematopoiesis	pubic arch
humerus	radius
ilium	range of motion
intercostal muscles	resorption
irritability	sacrum
isometric	scapula
isotonic	sinus
joint	sternum
kyphosis	symphysis pubis
lateral malleolus	tendons
ligaments	thorax
lordosis	tibia
malleolus	ulna
marrow	vertebral column
maxilla	

KEY POINTS

- The skeleton is the living framework of the human body.
- The four main types of bone are long, short, flat, and irregular.
- Red bone marrow is found in the ends of long bones, in the bodies of vertebrae, and in flat bones. Red bone marrow is responsible for hematopoiesis, or the manufacture of red blood cells, white blood cells, and platelets.
- Joints, bursae, ligaments, and cartilage are responsible for connecting skeletal parts, allowing for movement of skeletal parts, and protecting the skeleton from injury upon impact.
- The two divisions of the skeleton are the axial skeleton, which contains the bones of the center section, and the appendicular skeleton, which contains the bones of the extremities.

- Three main types of muscle tissue are skeletal (voluntary), smooth (involuntary), and cardiac. Muscle movements are voluntary or involuntary.
- The diaphragm and intercostal muscles are the primary muscles of respiration.
- Ossification is the process by which bones become hardened through an increase in calcified tissue. Bones change in size and composition during one's lifetime.
- Muscles work in groups that have opposing actions. When one muscle contracts, the other relaxes.
- Most of the heat in the body is generated from the cellular muscle activity of ATP and oxygen.
- The musculoskeletal system loses its flexibility and strength as people age.

■ Teaching–Learning Strategies

CLASSROOM

1. Ask the students to define the following terms and abbreviations:

ROM	sacrum
gait	scapula
osteoclast	periosteum
articulation	radius
hematopoiesis	kyphosis
osteocyte	joint
humerus	ligaments
bursae	lordosis
carpal	muscle tone
cartilage	marrow
contractility	ossification
diaphysis	tibia
elasticity	tendons
femur	thorax
irritability	tibia
intercostal muscles	symphysis pubis
patella	osteoclast
pelvis	ulna
clavicle	skull
coccyx	vertebral column
epiphysis	metatarsals
extensibility	phalanges
isometric	carpals
isotonic	hyoid

Write the students' responses on the chalkboard or on an overhead transparency.

2. Labeling exercises: Ask the students to label the:
   a. Major bones of the human skeleton
   b. Bones of the skull
   c. Diagram of a long bone
   d. Bones of the thorax
   e. Bones of the pelvis
   f. Bones of the hand and foot
   g. Muscles of the body

3. Show the videotape(s) *The Skeletal System* (29 minutes) and *The Muscular System* (25 minutes; available from Nimco, Inc., P.O. Box 9, 102 Highway 81 North, Calhoun, KY 42327). After viewing the videotapes, open the class for questions and discussion.

CLINICAL

1. In the learning laboratory, assign pairs of students to perform a skeletal and muscular assessment on each other. Ask students to document their findings on a piece of paper.

2. In the clinical setting, assign students to clients in various age groups to perform a musculoskeletal assessment. Ask the students to document their findings on a separate piece of paper or in the client's record. Ask students to share their findings with the larger group.

3. In the clinical setting, assign students to review the client's record and document the physician's orders on a piece of paper. Ask the students to share their findings with the larger group.

4. Assign a small number of students to a rehabilitation setting or physical therapy setting to observe clients with musculoskeletal disorders and their therapies. Ask the students to share their observations with the larger group.

ADDITIONAL RESOURCE

The Human Anatomy Online website contains information on skeletal and muscular systems: *www.innerbody.com/htm/body.html.*

CHAPTER 19

The Nervous System

LEARNING OBJECTIVES

1. Name and describe the three parts of a neuron.

2. Explain how the axon, dendrite, and neurotransmitter work together to transmit impulses.

3. Give an example of a sensory, motor, and interneuron impulse.

4. List the primary functions of each of the four cerebral lobes.

5. Explain how an injury to the cerebellum might present in an individual. Describe two nursing implications related to alteration in the cerebellum.

6. Identify the role of the limbic system in maintaining a person's level of awareness.

7. State the function of the medulla oblongata, pons, and midbrain. What two nursing considerations would be appropriate for the client with a dysfunction of the brain stem?

8. List the two functions of the spinal cord. Compare and contrast temporary and permanent paralysis and state two nursing assessments that would be performed for a client with paralysis.

9. Identify the three meninges.

10. Describe the function of the cerebrospinal fluid. What signs or symptoms might a client have who is experiencing a CSF leak?

11. List the 12 cranial nerves and the function of each.

12. List three functions of spinal nerves.

13. Compare and contrast the function of the parasympathetic and sympathetic nervous system.

14. Explain what is meant by the action potential of a nerve cell.

15. List three reflexes commonly tested in adults and three reflexes commonly tested in infants. Perform these assessments in nursing skills lab.

NEW TERMINOLOGY

action potential	neuroglia
afferent	neurology
axon	neuron
brain stem	neurotransmitter
cerebellum	occipital lobe
cerebrum	parasympathetic
cranial nerves	parietal lobe
decussation	peripheral nervous system
dendrites	plexus
effectors	pons
efferent	receptors
frontal lobe	reflex
glial cells	reflex arc
hypothalamus	spinal cord
interneuron	spinal nerves
limbic system	sympathetic
medulla	synapse
meninges	temporal lobe
midbrain	thalamus
myelin sheath	vagus nerve
nerve	ventricle

KEY POINTS

- The primary functions of the nervous system are communication and control.
- The two types of cells of the nervous system are the neuron and the neuroglia.
- A neuron consists of a cell body, axon, and dendrites.
- The central nervous system consists of the brain and the spinal cord.
- The four cerebral lobes are the frontal, parietal, temporal, and occipital. The frontal lobe is responsible for higher mental processes. The parietal lobe is responsible for speech and some sensory input. The temporal lobes are responsible

for smell, hearing, and some memory. The occipital lobe is responsible for vision.

- The thalamus is responsible for mood and strong emotions. The hypothalamus regulates many body functions such as temperature, thirst, hunger, urination, swallowing, and the sleep-wake cycle. The cerebellum is responsible for muscle control.
- The brain stem is made up of the midbrain, pons, and medulla. The midbrain functions as a reflex center. The pons contains nerve tracts and carrier messages between the cerebrum and medulla. The pons also is responsible for respirations. The medulla contains centers for vital body functions such as heart rate, vasomotor tone, and respirations.
- The two functions of the spinal cord include conducting impulses to and from the brain and acting as a reflex center.
- The three meninges include the dura mater, arachnoid, and pia mater.
- The spinal nerves are divided into 8 cervical pairs, 12 thoracic pairs, 5 lumbar pairs, 5 sacral pairs, and 1 coccygeal pair.
- The autonomic nervous system is divided into the sympathetic and parasympathetic divisions. The sympathetic system prepares individuals for emergencies. The parasympathetic system maintains normal body functions under regular conditions.
- The three types of neurons are sensory (afferent), motor (efferent), and interneurons (integrators). Sensory neurons carry information to the brain. Motor neurons carry information away from the brain. Interneurons respond to viscera.

■Teaching–Learning Strategies

CLASSROOM

1. Ask students to define the following terms and abbreviations:

ANS	hypothalamus
CNS	frontal nerve
CSF	midbrain
kg	interneuron
PNS	nerve
EEG	receptors
dexterity	pons medulla
action potential	reflex
dendrites	reflex arc
neuron	spinal cord
afferent	parietal lobe
efferent	neuroglia

cerebrum	spinal nerves
cranial nerves	plexus
decussation	meninges
myelin sheath	neurology
cerebellum	limbic system
axon	

Write the students' responses on the chalkboard or on an overhead transparency.

2. *Labeling exercises*: Ask the students to label the
   a. Structure of unmyelinated and myelinated neurons
   b. The human brain
   c. The autonomic nervous system and organs affected

3. Show the videotape *The Autonomic Nervous System* (1993; 28 minutes; available from Nimco, Inc., P.O. Box 9, 102 Highway 81 North, Calhoun, KY 42327). After viewing the videotape, open the class for questions and discussion.

4. Demonstrate the testing of various reflexes.

5. Outline the effects of aging on the nervous system.

CLINICAL

1. In the learning laboratory, demonstrate the testing of the 12 cranial nerves. Ask the students to join in pairs and practice testing each other's cranial nerves and reflexes. Ask the students to write their findings on a piece of paper and share their findings with the larger group.

2. In the clinical setting, assign students to a client. Ask the students to assess the client's reflexes and cranial nerve function. Ask the students to document their findings on a separate piece of paper or in the client's record. Ask the students to share their findings with the larger group.

3. In the clinical setting, ask the students to write the physician's orders on a separate piece of paper and share these findings with the larger group.

4. In the clinical setting, assign students to work with a nurse who is caring for a client with a nervous system deviation or disorder. Ask the

students to share their nursing care plans with the larger group.

ADDITIONAL RESOURCES

Human Anatomy Online has a website that has a link to the nervous system: *www.innerbody.com/htm/body.html*.

National Institute of Neurologic Disorders and Stroke is part of the National Institutes of Health and has a website with links to various resources: *www.ninds.nih.gov/*. In addition, there is an alphabetical listing of disorders with links to information related to these disorders at *www.ninds.nih.gov/health_and_medical/disorder_index.htm*

Neuroscience for Kids has information on the brain and spinal cord: *faculty.washington.edu/chudler/neurok.html*.

Society for Neuroscience also provides information about disorders and diseases on its website: *http://www.apu.sfn.org/briefings/info_dis_disease.html*.

CHAPTER 20

The Endocrine System

LEARNING OBJECTIVES

1. Differentiate between exocrine and endocrine glands.

2. Name three general functions of the endocrine system.

3. Describe the relationship between the hypothalamus and the pituitary gland.

4. Name and state the function of the hormones of the anterior and posterior pituitary gland.

5. Discuss the hormones responsible for calcium balance.

6. Describe the hormones involved in "fight or flight," and give three examples of their response during an emergency.

7. Explain the function of the thyroid hormones.

8. Locate the adrenal glands and describe the function of the mineralocorticoids and glucocorticoids. What are four nursing implications in caring for a patient taking a glucocorticoid?

9. Discuss the location of insulin secretion and explain how insulin and glucagon regulate blood sugar. What signs or symptoms might be seen in a client who lacks insulin production?

10. Identify the glands of reproduction and the sex hormones they produce.

11. Discuss negative feedback as it relates to the endocrine system.

12. Describe two functions of prostaglandins.

13. Describe four effects of aging on the endocrine system.

NEW TERMINOLOGY

adenohypophysis	hypothalamus
adrenal glands	insulin
corticosteroids	islets of Langerhans
endocrine glands	mineralocorticoids
erythropoietin	neurohypophysis
exocrine glands	parathyroids
gland	pineal gland
glucagons	pituitary gland
glucocorticoids	prostaglandins
glycogen	thymus
hormones	thyroid gland

KEY POINTS

- Endocrine glands secrete hormones to target tissues through the circulatory system. Exocrine glands secrete hormones into ducts. Hormones are chemical regulators that integrate and coordinate body activities.
- The nervous system tissue of the hypothalamus controls the pituitary gland. The many hormones of the anterior and posterior pituitary lobes have widespread effects on the body.
- The thyroid is responsible for controlling the body's rate of metabolism.
- The parathyroids regulate the amount of calcium and phosphorus in the blood.
- The adrenal medulla secretes hormones that mimic the action of the sympathetic nervous system. These hormones are active in emergencies or stressful situations.
- The adrenal cortex makes the three types of steroid compounds from cholesterol: mineralocorticoids, glucocorticoids, and sex hormones. These sex hormones supplement those secreted by the gonads, the glands of reproduction.
- As an endocrine gland, the pancreas secretes insulin, which lowers blood sugar, and glucagons, which raises blood sugar.

- The thymus secretes hormones that play a role in cellular immunity.
- Melatonin, the hormone secreted by the pineal gland, helps regulate the sleep/wake cycle.
- Prostaglandins are hormone-like substances. Their effects are localized to the area in which they are produced. They influence blood pressure, respiration, digestion, and reproduction.
- The endocrine system has close relationships with other body systems.
- Negative feedback mechanisms influence hormonal blood levels. Hormones are specific to target tissues and act in a "lock-and-key" fashion.
- Reduced hormonal production occurs as part of the normal aging process.

▪Teaching–Learning Strategies

CLASSROOM

1. Ask the students to define the following terms and abbreviations:

ACTH	GnRH
ADH	GHIH
ANP	pituitary gland
CRH	glucagons
FSH	thymus
HCG	thyroid gland
ICSH	adrenal glands
GH	gland
LH	pineal gland
MIH	pancreas
MSH	hormones
PIH	hypothalamus
PRH	insulin
PRL	islets of Langerhans
PTH	corticosteroid
TSH	endocrine glands
T_3	exocrine glands
T_4	

Write the students' responses on the chalkboard or on an overhead transparency.

2. Labeling exercises: Ask the students to label the main hormone-secreting glands.

3. Ask the students to compare and contrast the endocrine and exocrine glands. Write the students' responses on the chalkboard or on an overhead transparency.

4. Assign pairs of students to a specific gland. Ask each pair of students to identify the hormone(s) secreted and the action(s) of the specific gland.

CLINICAL

1. In the clinical setting, assign each student to work with a nurse who is caring for clients with endocrine disorders. Ask each student to review the client's record and document laboratory findings related to the endocrine system. Ask each student to share these findings with the larger group.

2. In the clinical setting assign a small group of students to observe in an operating room setting, where surgical procedures are performed on clients with endocrine disorders (e.g., thyroidectomy). Ask the students to share their findings with the larger group.

3. In the clinical setting where there are clients with endocrine disorders, assign each student to a specific client. Ask each student to write the physician's orders on a separate piece of paper and to share these findings with the larger group.

4. In the learning laboratory, show the videotape *Pathophysiology of Diabetes* (1997; 20 minutes; available from Lippincott Williams & Wilkins, 530 Walnut Street, Philadelphia, PA 19106). After viewing the videotape, open the class for questions and discussion.

5. In the learning laboratory, assign students to practice using insulin therapy equipment.

ADDITIONAL RESOURCES

The Altruis Biomedical Network has a website related to endocrinology. The site discusses several hormones, including corticosteroids, prostaglandins, and testosterone:*www.e-hormone.com/.*

Human Anatomy Online has a website related to all body systems. Click on the icon for the endocrine system: *www.innerbody.com/htm/body.html.*

CHAPTER 21

The Sensory System

LEARNING OBJECTIVES

1. Name the five senses. Where are the receptors for each? What part of the brain interprets the stimulus for each sense?

2. Describe the sclera, the choroid, cornea, iris, conjunctiva, the lacrimal gland, and the retina. Discuss their functions.

3. Differentiate between aqueous humor and vitreous humor.

4. Which cranial nerves are responsible for the blink reflex, pupillary changes, visualization, and pain sensation in the eye?

5. Differentiate between myopia and hyperopia and give an example of each.

6. Identify the anatomic landmark that divides the outer from the middle ear. Which divides the middle from the inner ear?

7. Trace the path of light rays as they enter the eye and focus on the retina.

8. Trace the path of sound waves through the ear.

9. Explain how cerumen, the ossicles, and eustachian tube work in protecting the ear.

10. Discuss how the organs of the ear work to provide a sense of balance.

11. What are the four types of taste buds? Locate where they are found on the tongue.

12. Describe six effects of aging on the sensory system.

13. Discuss the nursing implications for a client with decreased vision.

14. Discuss the nursing implications for a client with a loss of taste and smell.

15. Describe how would you go about teaching a client about a certain medical disorder, medication, or procedure if the client has presbycusis.

NEW TERMINOLOGY

accommodation	olfaction
aqueous humor	optic disk
auricle	orbit
cerumen	organ of Corti
cochlea	ossicles
cones	pinna
conjunctiva membrane	presbycusis
cornea	presbyopia
eustachian tube	proprioceptors
hyperopia	pupil
incus	retina
iris	rods
labyrinth	sclera
lacrimal glands	semicircular canals
lens	stapes
malleus	tympanic membrane
membranous labyrinth	vertigo
myopia	vitreous humor

KEY POINTS

- The five senses are seeing, hearing, tasting, smelling, and touching.
- The eye is the organ of vision. It has many protective mechanisms. Light rays travel through several structures of the eye before focusing on the retina.
- The eyeball has three major layers of tissue: sclera and cornea, choroids layer, and retina.
- Several cranial nerves are involved in eye functioning.
- Six extraocular muscles control eye movements.
- The three parts of the ear are the external, middle, and inner ears.
- The middle ear is responsible for the transmission of sound.
- The semicircular canals of the inner ear are responsible for balance.
- Taste buds are responsible for the perceptions of sweet, salty, sour, and bitter.
- Receptors for smell are located in the upper nasal cavity.
- Receptors for the sense of touch are called tactile receptors.

- Proprioceptors are located in muscles, tendons, and joints.
- Referred pain is perceived in a place other than where it originates.
- The temporal, parietal, occipital, and cerebellar areas of the brain are responsible for interpreting sensory stimuli.

■Teaching–Learning Strategies

CLASSROOM

1. Ask the students to define the following terms and abbreviations:

lacrimal glands	auricle
proprioceptors	hyperopia
aqueous humor	iris
retina	myopia
lens	cones
presbyopia	cornea
sclera	olfaction
cochlea	Eustachian tube
rods	ossicles
pupil	optic disk
cerumen	vertigo
nystagmus	semicircular canals

Write the students' responses on the chalkboard or on an overhead transparency.

2. Labeling exercises: Ask the students to label the following:
   a. The right eye with its lacrimal glands and ducts
   b. The lateral view of the eye and its appendages
   c. The ear
   d. Surface of the tongue

3. Show the videotape *The Sensory System* (28 minutes; available from Nimco, Inc., P.O. Box 9, 102 Highway 81 North, Calhoun, KY 42327).

After viewing the videotape, open the class for questions and discussion.

CLINICAL

1. In the learning laboratory, show students models or charts of the eye, ear, and tongue. Ask the students to identify the major structures. Ask students to join in pairs and assess each others' sensory system. Ask the students to write their findings on a piece of paper and share their findings with the larger group.

2. In the clinical setting, assign students to clients who have disorders of the sensory system. Ask students to review and record the physician's orders from the client's record (chart) and ask the students to share their findings with the larger clinical group.

3. Assign students to interview an older adult. Ask the students to interview the client about the effects of aging on the sensory system. Ask students to record their findings in a summary paper.

4. In the clinical setting, assign students to work with a nurse who is caring for clients with sensory disorders. After this experience, ask the students to share their observations and nursing care plans with the larger group.

ADDITIONAL RESOURCES

Eye anatomy and conditions: *www.eyemdlink.com*
The National Institute of Neurologic Disorders and Strokes has an alphabetical listing of disorders: *www.ninds.nig.gov/health__and__medical/disorder__index. htm.*
The Society for Neuroscience website contains information on sleep, pain, and vestibular disorders: *www.sfn.org/briefings/info__dis__disease.html.*
Study Web contains information on anatomy and biology: *www.studyweb.com/.*

CHAPTER 22

The Cardiovascular System

LEARNING OBJECTIVES

1. Differentiate between the endocardium, myocardium, pericardium and epicardium.

2. Describe the chambers of the heart and locate them on an anatomical model. State and locate on an anatomical model the vessels that enter and exit these chambers.

3. Define and describe the function of the atrioventricular valves, semilunar valves, chordae tendineae, and papillary muscles.

4. On a chart or model, trace the path of blood through both sides of the heart using correct terminology.

5. List, locate, and describe the structure and function of the coronary arteries that supply the heart tissue (myocardium) with blood. Explain the purpose of collateral circulation.

6. Compare and contrast arteries, capillaries, and veins and describe the function of each.

7. Describe the path of an electrical impulse through the conduction system of the heart. Describe the purpose of this electrical activity.

8. Explain what creates the normal heart sounds, S_1 and S_2, and note where each of these sounds is best heard.

9. Define cardiac output and describe the factors that regulate it.

10. Define blood pressure and differentiate between systolic and diastolic pressures.

11. Identify factors that affect the regulation of blood pressure.

12. State four changes in the cardiovascular system caused by aging. Discuss the nursing implications for each.

NEW TERMINOLOGY

afterload
aorta
aortic valve
apex
atria
bicuspid valve
collateral circulation
coronary sinus
diastole
endocardium
epicardium
ischemia
microcirculation
mitral valve
myocardium
pericardial fluid
pericardium
preload
pulmonic valve
pulse
pulse pressure
semilunar valve
septum
systole
tricuspid valve

KEY POINTS

• The cardiovascular system consists of the heart and blood vessels.
• The heart is a strong, muscular pump that lies between the lungs in the mediastinum.
• The heart wall has three layers: endocardium, myocardium, and epicardium. The epicardium also is the innermost layer of the surrounding pericardium that cushions and protects the heart.
• The septum divides the heart into right and left halves. The heart is further divided into four chambers: two superior atria and two inferior ventricles.
• The valves of the heart allow unidirectional blood flow through the heart.
• The principal arteries that supply the heart muscle itself with blood are the right and left coronary arteries.
• Arteries, capillaries, and veins carry blood through the body.
• The conduction system of the heart consists of unique tissue specializing in the formation, transmission, and coordination of electrical impulses that stimulate the heart to beat.
• The normal "pacemaker" of the heart is the SA node.
• A cardiac cycle lasts less than 1 second and consists of the contraction (systole) and relaxation (diastole) of both atria, followed by both ventricles.
• Events in the cardiac cycle create normal, and sometimes extra, heart sounds.

- Cardiac output is the amount of blood the ventricles pump out in 1 minute. The formula for calculating cardiac output is CO = SV (stroke volume) × HR (heart rate). Normally, cardiac output equals 4 to 6 L/min.
- Blood pressure is the force blood exerts against the walls of the blood vessels. Systolic blood pressure is the force during ventricular contraction. Diastolic blood pressure is the force during ventricular relaxation.
- The nervous, endocrine, cardiovascular, and urinary systems work together to regulate blood pressure.
- Separating normal physiologic changes of the cardiovascular system in older adults is difficult because changes often are interrelated with heredity, lifestyle, habits, and co-existing diseases or disorders.

■ Teaching–Learning Strategies

CLASSROOM

1. Ask the students to define the following terms and abbreviations:

AV	apex
BP	diastole
CO	atria
HR	bicuspid
LAD	systole
LCA	endocardium
LCX	epicardium
LMCA	myocardium
RCA	pulse
SA	apex
SV	preload
SVR	septum
afterload	pacemaker
aorta	semilunar valves

Write the students' responses on the chalkboard or on an overhead transparency.

2. Labeling exercises: Ask the students to label the:
   a. Heart and great vessels
   b. Coronary arteries and veins
   c. Major systemic arteries and pulse points
   d. Conduction system of the heart

3. Show the videotape *Human Cardiovascular System* (28 minutes; available from Nimco, Inc., P.O. Box 9, 102 Highway 81 North, Calhoun, KY 42327). After viewing the videotape, open the class for questions and discussion.

CLINICAL

1. Ask the students to view the interactive videodisk *An Introduction to Cardiovascular Examination* by C.V. Mosby, Mirror Systems, Cambridge, Massachusetts. After the students have seen the program, open the class for questions and discussion.

2. Demonstrate the various structures of the heart and major arteries with charts or models. Ask students to identify major structures, arteries, and pulse points. Demonstrate the technique of auscultation of heart sounds. Ask students to join in pairs and practice auscultation on each other.

3. In the clinical setting, assign students to work with a nurse who is caring for clients with cardiovascular disorders. Ask the students to locate the client's pulses and auscultate the client's heart sounds. Ask students to write their findings in the client's record or on a separate piece of paper. Ask students to share their findings with the larger group.

4. Assign a small group of students to a diagnostic center for cardiovascular disorders or to an operating room setting where cardiac surgery is performed. Ask students to share their observations with the larger group.

5. Assign students to perform a cardiac assessment on an older adult. Ask students to summarize their findings in a one- to two-page paper. Ask the students to share their findings with the larger group.

ADDITIONAL RESOURCES

The Altruis Biomedical Network has a website with cardiovascular information, including links to the topics of heart and heart disease, vascular disease, blood pressure, and arteries/veins: *www.e-cardiovascular.net/*.

American Heart Association, website: *www.americanheart.org/*

Human Anatomy Online has information on the cardiovascular system at its website: *www.innerbody.com/html/body.html*.

National Heart, Lung and Blood Institute, National Institutes of Health, website: *www.nhlbi.nih.gov*

CHAPTER 23

The Hematologic and Lymphatic Systems

LEARNING OBJECTIVES

1. Describe the principal functions of the blood and its mechanisms for maintaining homeostasis.

2. Identify the four plasma proteins and their chief functions.

3. Outline the structure and functions of the red blood cells, white blood cells, and platelets.

4. Discuss the importance of chemotaxis and phagocytosis in fighting foreign invaders.

5. Describe the mechanism of blood clotting.

6. Identify the four blood groups and explain Rh. Discuss what components contribute to the color of blood.

7. Name the universal recipient and universal donor. Explain why they are so named.

8. Illustrate pulmonary and systemic circulation routes.

9. Describe lymphatic circulation and the filtration role of the lymph nodes.

10. Describe the circle of Willis and the blood–brain barrier, and state their functions.

11. Explain where blood from the digestive organs and spleen travels before returning to the heart.

12. Describe what occurs, regarding the blood, in the digestive organs and spleen.

13. Discuss at least three normal changes in the hematologic and lymphatic systems caused by aging.

NEW TERMINOLOGY

agglutination
albumin
anastomose
coagulation
crossmatching
embolus
endocytosis
erythrocyte
fibrin
fibrinogen
globulin
hematopoiesis
hemorrhage
hemostasis
leukocyte

lymph
lymph nodes
lymphocyte
monocyte
phagocytosis
plasma
platelet
prothrombin
Rh factor
spleen
thrombin
thrombocyte
thrombus
tonsil

KEY POINTS

- Blood is composed of plasma and formed elements.
- The function of the hematologic system is transportation, regulation, and protection.
- The major elements of the blood are RBCs, WBCs, and platelets.
- Hematopoiesis, formation of blood cells, originates in stem cells in red bone marrow.
- Plasma is 90% water. The remaining 10% is composed of proteins, salts, nutrients, wastes, gases, hormones, and enzymes.
- Erythrocytes, or RBCs, are the most numerous of the blood cells. Each RBC contains hemoglobin, which is responsible for carrying oxygen.
- All WBCs fight infection. Each of the five types has different mechanisms to combat invaders.
- Platelets and numerous clotting factors must react in sequence before clotting can occur.

- Hemorrhage usually is thought of as the loss of a considerable amount of blood. Hemostasis refers to the stoppage of bleeding.
- The ABO and Rh blood groups are inherited combinations of antigens and antibodies.
- Lymph tissues filter blood, destroy pathogens, and develop antibodies against antigens.
- Lymphatic organs include the tonsils, spleen, and thymus.
- The pulmonary circulation allows blood to be oxygenated for distribution in the systemic circulation.
- The largest circulatory route is the systemic circulation, which transports oxygen, nutrients, and wastes to and from all body cells.
- Several arteries come together to form the circle of Willis. This arterial circle helps to maintain and protect cerebral blood flow to the brain.
- The blood–brain barrier selectively determines what substances will enter the brain from the blood. Its purpose is to prevent harmful substances from entering the brain.
- The hepatic portal circulation detours venous blood from the abdominal organs to the liver before returning it to the heart.
- Lymph drains interstitial fluid into lymphatic vessels and returns the fluid back to the veins.

■ Teaching–Learning Strategies

CLASSROOM

1. Ask the students to define the following terms and abbreviations:

B cell	hematopoiesis
B lymphocyte	fibrinogen
CO$_2$	leukocytes
Hgb/Hb	lymph
Ig	lymph nodes
O$_2$	monocytes
RBC	plasma
Rh	spleen
T cell	prothrombin
WBC	tonsils
agglutination	hemostasis
albumin coagulation	stem cells
erythrocytes	marrow
hemorrhage	

Write the students' responses on the chalkboard or on an overhead transparency.

2. Labeling exercise: Ask the students to label the
   a. Types of WBCs
   b. Lymphatic system
   c. Hepatic-portal circulation

3. Show the videotape *The Lymphatic and Reticuloendothelial System* (25 minutes; available from Nimco, Inc., P.O. Box 9, 102 Highway 81 North, Calhoun, KY 42327). After viewing the videotape, open the class for questions and discussion.

CLINICAL

1. Demonstrate the various structures of the lymphatic system with charts or models. Ask students to identify major structures of the lymphatic system.

2. In the clinical setting, assign students to work with a nurse who is caring for clients with lymphatic or hematologic disorders. Ask the students to locate the various lymphatic glands and assess for edema. Ask students to write their findings in the client's record or on a separate piece of paper. Ask students to share their findings with the larger group.

3. Assign a small group of students to visit a clinical laboratory where blood is typed and crossmatched. Ask the students to interview a clinical laboratory employee about precautions that are taken when blood is typed and crossmatched. Ask the students to share their observations with the larger group.

4. In the clinical setting, assign students to a client with a hematologic or lymphatic disorder. Ask the students to review the physician's orders and write these orders on a separate piece of paper. Ask the students to review the client's laboratory blood studies (e.g., type and Rh) and record their findings. Ask the students to share their findings with the larger group.

ADDITIONAL RESOURCES

Human Anatomy Online has a link with information on the lymphatic system: *www.innerbody.com/htm/body.html*

CHAPTER 24

The Immune System

LEARNING OBJECTIVES

1. Explain lymphocytes and where they are produced.

2. Differentiate between B cells and T cells.

3. Name the five categories of antibodies and describe two nursing implications related to a lack of or decrease in antibody production.

4. Differentiate between nonspecific and specific immunity.

5. Differentiate between naturally acquired active and passive immunity and artificially acquired active and passive immunity, and give an example of each.

6. Describe the process of antigen–antibody-mediated immunity.

7. Explain how the "lock-and-key" concept applies to the antigen–antibody complex.

8. List the three mechanisms antibodies use to destroy antigens.

9. Describe two effects of aging on the immune system.

NEW TERMINOLOGY

acquired immunity	immunization
antibody-mediated immunity	inborn immunity
artificially acquired immunity	macrophage
B cells/B lymphocytes	naturally acquired immunity
cell-mediated immunity	nonspecific immunity
complement fixation	specific immunity
gamma globulin	T cells/T lymphocytes
humoral immunity	thymus
immunity	vaccine

KEY POINTS

- Immunity is the specific resistance to disease that involves the production of a specific lymphocyte or antibody against a specific antigen.

- Both B cells and T cells derive from stem cells in the bone marrow.
- B cells go on to mature in the bone marrow, whereas T cells complete their maturation and develop immunocompetence in the thymus gland.
- Antigens are substances the immune system recognizes as foreign.
- An antibody is a protein that combines specifically with the antigen that triggers its production.
- Humoral immunity refers to destruction of antigens by antibodies.
- Cell-mediated immunity refers to destruction of antigens by T cells.
- Exposure to disease-causing organisms over one's lifetime stimulates the process of acquired immunity.
- Humoral or antigen–antibody-mediated immunity protects the body against circulating disease-producing antigens and bacteria.
- Antibodies use several mechanisms to destroy antigens: neutralizing toxins, facilitating phagocytosis, and complement fixation.

■Teaching–Learning Strategies

CLASSROOM

1. Ask the students to define the following terms and abbreviations:

AB	TF
Ig	THF
IgG	antigen
IgM	immunity gamma globulin
IgA	macrophage
IgE	inborn immunity
IgD	artificially acquired immunity

Write the students' responses on the chalkboard or on an overhead transparency.

2. Show the videotape *The Immune System* (28 minutes; available from Nimco, Inc., P.O. Box 9, 102 Highway 81 North, Calhoun, KY 42327). After viewing the videotape, open the class for questions and discussion.

3. Invite a nurse who cares for clients with compromised immune systems (e.g., clients with cancer) to visit the class and present the role of the nurse in caring for such clients. After the presentation, open the class for questions and discussion.

CLINICAL

1. In the clinical setting, assign students to work with a nurse who is caring for clients with compromised immune systems. Ask the students to indicate what precautions must be taken when caring for clients with compromised immune systems. Ask students to share their findings and observations with the larger group.

2. In the clinical setting, assign students to a client with a compromised immune system. Ask the students to review the client's record and document the physician's orders on a separate piece of paper. Ask students to review the client's laboratory blood studies and record the client's laboratory values. Ask students to share their findings with the larger group.

3. Assign students to perform a physical assessment of an older adult. Assign students to interview the client about the effects of aging on the client's immune system. Ask students to summarize their findings in a one- to two-page paper. Ask the students to share their findings with the larger group.

ADDITIONAL RESOURCES

The Cells Alive website has a "cell gallery" with information on antibody production and anatomy of a splinter, showing the inflammatory process: *www.cellsalive.com/*.

Human Anatomy Online has a link with information about the lymphatic system: *www.innerbody.com/htm/body.html*.

Indiana State University has a website with information on altered immune responses *www.web.indstate.edu/nurs/mary/fluidlytecf/*

CHAPTER 25

The Respiratory System

LEARNING OBJECTIVES

1. Differentiate between internal and external respiration.

2. Describe the anatomic relationship between the larynx, trachea, and esophagus.

3. Name and describe four ways in which the respiratory system is protected.

4. Name the structures and diagram the path that air must travel in and out of the lungs.

5. Explain how inspiration and expiration occur.

6. Define pleura and describe its action.

7. Differentiate between TV, TLC, VC, IRV, and ERV. Discuss a possible cause for a decreased ERV, decreased TLC, or increased FRC and two nursing implications for each disorder.

8. Describe two regulators of breathing.

9. Describe how exchange of gases takes place in the lungs (pleura).

10. Describe two effects of aging on the respiratory system and state a nursing implication for each.

NEW TERMINOLOGY

alveolar ducts	mediastinum
alveolar sacs	nares
bronchi	nasopharynx
bronchioles	oropharynx
cellular respiration	parietal pleura
cilia	pharynx
diaphragm	pleura
dyspnea	pleural cavity
epiglottis	pleural space
eupnea	respiration
expiration	sinuses
external respiration	surfactant
inspiration	trachea
intercostal muscles	ventilation
internal respiration	visceral pleura
larynx	vocal cords
lungs	

KEY POINTS

- The pathway for external breathing is nose → pharynx → larynx → trachea → bronchi → bronchioles → alveoli (where oxygen is exchanged for carbon dioxide).
- The pharynx is divided into three areas: nasopharynx, oropharynx, and laryngopharynx.
- The trachea and esophagus are both located in the pharynx. The epiglottis is a protective flap that covers the trachea during swallowing to prevent foreign matter from entering the respiratory system.
- The pleura has two layers. One layer covers the lung and the other layer lines the chest wall. Serous fluid secreted by the pleura enables the lungs to move without pain or friction.
- External respiration is the exchange of gas at the lung level. Internal respiration is the exchange of gas at the cellular level.
- The various lung volumes and capacities describe the volume of air in the lungs (or left in the lungs) in relation to inspiration or expiration. These amounts can vary depending upon the gender of the client and respiratory disorders that the client may have.
- The pathway for oxygen distribution and carbon dioxide return (internal breathing) is alveoli → capillaries (hemoglobin combines with oxygen) → cells → capillaries (carbon dioxide exchange) → alveoli.
- Nasal hair, mucus, and cilia are protective structures of the respiratory system. Sneezing, coughing, and yawning are protective reflexes of the respiratory system.

■ Teaching–Learning Strategies

CLASSROOM

1. Ask the students to define the following terms and abbreviations:

CO	diaphragm
CO_2	epiglottis
ERV	dyspnea
H_2CO_3	inspiration
IRV	expiration
O_2	pleura
RV	sinuses
TLC	respiration
TV	surfactant
VC	trachea
pharynx	lungs
external respiration	mediastinum
bronchi	intercostal muscles
eupnea	cellular respiration
apnea	pleural cavity

Write the students' responses on the chalkboard or on an overhead transparency.

2. Show the videotape(s) *Thorax and Lungs* (20 minutes; available from Lippincott Williams & Wilkins, 530 Walnut Street, Philadelphia, PA 19106) and *The Respiratory System* (available from Nimco, Inc., P.O. Box 9, 102 Highway 81 North, Calhoun, KY 42327). After viewing the videotape(s), open the class for questions and discussion.

3. Invite a volunteer or a nurse who works with the American Lung Association to visit the class and present the role of the volunteer or nurse in prevention of respiratory disorders. After the presentation, open the class for questions and discussion.

CLINICAL

1. Demonstrate the various structures of the respiratory system with charts or models. Ask students to identify major structures related to respiration. Demonstrate the technique of auscultation of breath sounds. Ask students to join in pairs and practice auscultation of breath sounds on each other. Ask the students to document their findings on a separate piece of paper.

2. In the clinical setting, assign students to work with a nurse who is caring for clients with respiratory disorders. Ask the students to auscultate the client's breath sounds. Ask students to write their findings in the client's record or on a separate piece of paper. Ask students to share their findings with the larger group.

3. Assign a small group of students to a diagnostic center for respiratory disorders or to an operating room setting where lung/nasal surgery is performed. Ask students to share their observations with the larger group.

4. Assign students to perform a respiratory assessment on an older adult. Ask students to summarize their findings in a one- to two-page paper. Ask the students to share their findings with the larger group.

ADDITIONAL RESOURCES

American Lung Association, website: *www.lungusa.org*

Human Anatomy Online has information on the pulmonary system, including animation: *www.innerbody.com*

National Heart, Lung, Blood Institute, National Institute of Health, website: *www.nhlbi.nih.gov*

CHAPTER 26

The Digestive System

LEARNING OBJECTIVES

1. Trace the digestive pathway, naming the major organs of the gastrointestinal (GI) tract with their function.

2. Describe the following processes: mastication, deglutition, and peristalsis.

3. Explain the actions of hydrochloric acid (HCl), gastrin, intrinsic factor, cholecystokinin, and pancreatic juice.

4. Describe two functions of the pancreas and gallbladder in relation to digestion. Describe four functions of the liver.

5. Describe the physiology of digestion and absorption, including how nutrients are absorbed in the small intestine.

6. Identify and describe two major categories of metabolism.

7. Explain how the large intestine changes its contents into fecal material.

8. Describe three effects of aging on the digestive system.

NEW TERMINOLOGY

absorption	ingestion
alimentary canal	jejunum
bile	liver
bolus	mastication
cardiac sphincter	peristalsis
chyme	peritoneum
defecation	pyloric sphincter
deglutition	pylorus
digestion	rectum
duodenum	rugae
esophagus	saliva
gallbladder	salivation
ileum	villi

KEY POINTS

- Primary functions of the digestive system include digestion, absorption, and elimination.
- The digestive tract, or gastrointestinal (GI) tract, is a continuous tube beginning at the mouth and extending to the anus. It is open to the outside on both ends and is not sterile.
- The accessory organs of the digestive system include the liver, gallbladder, pancreas, and peritoneum.
- The two types of digestion are mechanical (chewing of food) and chemical (breakdown of food into usable form).
- The breaking down of food into smaller molecules is called digestion. The passage of these molecules into the circulation is called absorption.
- Most nutrient absorption occurs in the small intestine. The large intestine mainly reabsorbs water and produces vitamin K and some B complex vitamins.
- Metabolism is the total of all physical and chemical changes that occur in the body. It includes catabolism and anabolism.
- A variety of digestive changes in the elderly can place them at risk for fluid and electrolyte imbalance, dehydration, and malnutrition.

■ Teaching–Learning Strategies

CLASSROOM

1. Ask the students to define the following terms and abbreviations:

ATP	cardiac sphincter
CHO	digestion
GI	gallbladder
HCl	rectum
absorption	nutrients
alimentary canal	peritoneum
jejunum	tongue
liver	bony socket
mastication	bicuspids
esophagus	rugae

bile
bolus
chyme
defecation

pepsinogen
carbohydrates
gastric lipase

Write the students' responses on the chalkboard or on an overhead transparency.

2. Show the videotape *The Digestive System* (28 minutes; available from Nimco, Inc., P.O. Box 9, 102 Highway 81 North, Calhoun, KY 42327). After viewing the videotape, open the class for questions and discussion.

3. Ask students to form pairs. Assign each pair of students an organ of digestion and ask students to identify the specific enzyme secreted and its actions. Ask the students to share their findings with the larger group.

CLINICAL

1. Demonstrate the various structures of the digestive system with charts or models. Ask students to identify major structures related to digestion. Demonstrate the technique of auscultation of bowel sounds. Ask students to join in pairs and practice auscultation of bowel sounds on each other. Ask the students to document their findings on a separate piece of paper.

2. Ask the students to view the CD-ROM *The Human Digestive System* (1997; available from Insight Media, P.O. Box 621, New York, NY 10024). After viewing the disk, open the class for questions and discussion.

3. In the clinical setting, assign students to work with a nurse who is caring for clients with digestive disorders. Ask the students to auscultate the client's bowel sounds. Ask students to write

their findings in the client's record or on a separate piece of paper. Ask students to share their findings with the larger group.

4. Assign a small group of students to a diagnostic center for digestive disorders or to an operating room setting where surgery related to any of the digestive organs is performed. Ask students to share their observations with the larger group.

5. Assign students to perform a nutrition and digestion assessment on an older adult. Ask students to summarize their findings in a one- to two-page paper. Ask the students to share their findings with the larger group.

6. In the clinical setting, assign students to work with a nurse who is caring for clients with digestive disorders. Ask the students to identify the physician's orders, especially related to diet and fluids. Ask students to assist the client during meals. Ask students to write their findings in the client's record or on a separate piece of paper. Ask students to share their findings with the larger group.

ADDITIONAL RESOURCES

The Altruis Biomedical Network has a website for gastrointestinal information, including links to sites covering the topics of digestive glands, GI hormones, and digestion and absorption: *www.e-gastrointestinal.com*.

Human Anatomy Online has information on the digestive system: *www.innerbody.com/htm/body.html*.

CHAPTER 27

The Urinary System

LEARNING OBJECTIVES

1. Name the organs that constitute the urinary system.

2. Describe the anatomy and physiology of the nephron.

3. Explain how the urinary system influences homeostasis.

4. Identify and describe the function of the two hormones that kidneys secrete.

5. Explain how the kidney, ANP, and the RAA system affect red blood cells, blood pressure, water and electrolyte balance, acid–base balance, and vitamin D.

6. Describe blood supply to and from the kidneys.

7. Illustrate the pathway of waste products from the blood to the external environment.

8. Describe the formation of urine. Include the concepts of glomerular filtration, tubular reabsorption, and tubular secretion.

9. Describe the chemical differences between plasma, glomerular filtrate, and urine.

10. Compare and contrast micturition and incontinence.

11. List the characteristics and possible components of normal urine.

12. Describe three effects of aging on the urinary system and the nursing implications related to these effects.

NEW TERMINOLOGY

bladder	nephrons
Bowman's capsule	nocturia
calyces	renal cortex
convoluted tubule	renal medulla
filtration	ureter
glomerulus	urethra
kidney	urination
micturition	voiding

KEY POINTS

- The urinary system eliminates wastes, controls water volume, regulates electrolyte levels, maintains pH balance, activates vitamin D, and secretes rennin and erythropoietin.
- The kidneys lie behind the peritoneum (are retroperitoneal).
- Nephrons are the functional units of kidneys. Nephrons make urine; the rest of the urinary system expels it.
- Nephrons consist of renal corpuscles (glomeruli, Bowman's capsule) and renal tubules (proximal convoluted tubule, loop of Henle, distal convoluted tubule).
- Urine is 95% water and 5% solutes (salts, nitrogenous waste products, metabolites, hormones, toxins).
- Urine is formed by these three processes: glomerular filtration, tubular reabsorption, and tubular secretion.
- Micturition (voiding) is the release of urine; involuntary voiding is called urinary incontinence.
- As the body ages, the number of functional nephrons decreases.

■Teaching–Learning Strategies

CLASSROOM

1. Ask the students to define the following terms and abbreviations:

ADH	kidney
ANP	renal medulla
BUN	voiding
cm	urination
bladder	micturition
renal	glomerular filtration rate
glomerulus	nephrons
Bowman's capsule	urethra
filtration	catheterization
calyces	tubular reabsorption

Write the students' responses on the chalkboard or on an overhead transparency.

2. Show the videotape *The Urinary System* (29 minutes; available from Nimco, Inc., P.O. Box 9, 102 Highway 81 North, Calhoun, KY 42327). After viewing the videotape, open the class for questions and discussion.

3. Have students complete *Interactive Physiology: Urinary System* by A.D.A.M. Software, Inc., and Benjamin/Cummings Publishing Co. (2725 Sand Hill Road, Menlo Park, CA 94025).

4. Invite a nurse who cares for clients with disorders of the urinary system to visit the class and discuss the role of the nurse in caring for these clients. After the presentation, open the class for questions and discussion.

CLINICAL

1. Demonstrate the various structures of the urinary system with charts or models. Ask students to identify major structures. Demonstrate the procedure for measuring urinary output and have the students perform a return demonstration.

2. In the clinical setting, assign students to work with a nurse who is caring for clients with urinary disorders. Ask the students to measure the client's urinary output for the entire clinical period. Ask students to write their findings in the client's record or on a separate piece of paper. Ask students to share their findings with the larger group.

3. Assign a small group of students to a diagnostic center for urinary disorders or to an operating room setting where urinary surgery is performed. Ask students to share their observations with the larger group.

4. Assign students to locate one article related to the urinary system using the library or the Internet. Ask students to summarize their findings in a one- to two-page paper. Ask the students to share their findings with the larger group.

ADDITIONAL RESOURCES

The Altruis Biomedical Network has information on the kidneys, including links to the topics of urine, thirst, diuretics, and acid–base balance: *www.e-kidneys.net/*.

American Association of Nephrology Nurses, website: *www.anna.inurse.com*

Human Anatomy Online has information on the urinary system: *www.innerbody.com/html/body.html*.

National Kidney Foundation, website: *www.kidney.org*

CHAPTER 28

The Male Reproductive System

LEARNING OBJECTIVES

1. Name the three major classifications of hormones that influence the male reproductive system and their functions.

2. Identify the testes, penis, scrotum, and urinary meatus of the male in nursing skills lab and discuss their function.

3. Discuss the role of the epididymis, ductus deferens, and ejaculatory ducts in the male reproductive system.

4. Describe how sperm migrate through the reproductive system.

5. Describe the components of ejaculatory fluid and where they come from.

6. Explain how sperm and semen are deposited into the vagina for reproductive purposes.

7. State two effects of aging on the male reproductive system.

NEW TERMINOLOGY

androgens	interstitial cells
bulbourethral (Cowper's) glands	orgasm
	penis
circumcision	perineum
climacteric	prostate
copulation	puberty
ductus deferens	scrotum
ejaculation	semen
emission	seminal vesicles
erection	seminiferous tubules
foreskin	spermatozoa
glans penis	testes
gonads	testosterone

KEY POINTS

- Internal organs of the male reproductive system include the testes, ducts, and glands.
- External structures of the male reproductive system include the scrotum and penis.

- The ducts of the male reproductive system include the epididymis, ductus deferens, and ejaculatory ducts. Sperm mature in the epididymis, travel through the ductus deferens, and join other secretions in the ejaculatory duct before exiting the body.
- The scrotum is a sac that supports and protects the testes.
- The penis serves as a common passageway for both the urinary and reproductive systems.
- The male reproductive system is under the influence of hormones from the hypothalamus, pituitary, and gonads.
- Male hormones are called androgens. Testosterone is the main male androgen.
- In men, gonadotropic hormones stimulate the formation of sperm and the secretion of hormones from the sex organs.
- Ejaculatory fluid contains semen from the seminal vesicles, alkaline secretions from the prostate, and mucus from the bulbourethral glands.
- Sperm cells are called spermatozoa and are stored in the ductus deferens where they combine with semen.
- During copulation, the penis becomes firm in order to penetrate the vagina. The urethra within the penis serves as a passageway for sperm and semen during ejaculation.

■ Teaching–Learning Strategies

CLASSROOM

1. Ask the students to define the following terms and abbreviations:

FSH	emission
ICSH	ejaculation
androgens	prostate
hormones	puberty
erection	semen
scrotum	spermatozoa
testes	orgasm
Cowper's glands	testosterone
circumcision	epididymis
climacteric	inguinal canal
copulation	spermatic cord
ductus deferens	

Write the students' responses on the chalkboard or on an overhead transparency.

2. Show the videotape *The Reproductive System* (27 minutes; available from Nimco, Inc., P.O. Box 9, 102 Highway 81 North, Calhoun, KY 42327). After viewing the videotape, open the class for questions and discussion.

3. Show the videotape *The Father Factor: Paternally Caused Infertility* (53 minutes; available from Films for the Humanities and Sciences, P.O. Box 2053, Princeton, NJ 08543-2053). After viewing the videotape, open the class for questions and discussion.

4. Ask a nurse or an urologist who works with male clients with reproductive disorders to visit the class and present the role of the nurse in caring for these clients. After the presentation, open the class for questions and discussion.

CLINICAL

1. Demonstrate the various structures of the male reproductive system with charts or models. Ask students to identify major structures.

2. In the clinical setting, assign students to work with a nurse who is caring for clients with reproductive disorders for the clinical period. Ask the students to review the physician's orders and laboratory studies (e.g., sperm analysis) and write these on a separate piece of paper. Ask the students to share their findings with the larger group.

3. Role play a scenario and practice communication skills. Ask one student to volunteer to play the role of a male client who is impotent and ask the other student to play the role of the nurse. After the role-playing exercise, ask students for comments and feedback.

ADDITIONAL RESOURCES

The Altruis Biomedical Network has two links to topics associated with the male reproductive system. The first is the urogenital system, including anatomy, ejaculation, erection, and common disorders and sexually transmitted diseases: *www.urogenital.com/*. The second site has information on male hormones: *www.e-hormone.com/*.

Human Anatomy Online has information on the male reproductive system at *www.innerbody.com/htm/body.html.*

CHAPTER 29

The Female Reproductive System

LEARNING OBJECTIVES

1. Name the major hormones that influence the female reproductive system.

2. Describe the functions of the ovaries, uterus, clitoris, and vagina.

3. Explain the role of the mammary glands in the reproductive process.

4. Describe the function of LH, FSH, and progesterone in the female reproductive system.

5. Discuss the process of oocyte maturation and ovulation.

6. List the three phases of the ovarian cycle and what occurs during each phase.

7. List the three phases of the uterine cycle and what occurs during each phase.

8. Discuss menopause and the physical changes that accompany it.

9. Identify two effects of the aging process on the female reproductive system and the nursing implications for each.

NEW TERMINOLOGY

cervix	menstruation
clitoris	mons pubis
endometrium	oocyte
estrogens	ova
fallopian tubes	ovaries
fimbriae	oviducts
gonadotropic hormones	ovulation
hymen	perineum
labia majora	progesterone
labia minora	uterus
mammary glands	vagina
menarche	vulva
menopause	zygote

KEY POINTS

- Internal organs of the female reproductive system include the ovaries, oviducts, uterus, and vagina.
- External organs of the female reproductive system include the vulva and breasts.
- The egg cell is called an oocyte. Maturation begins in the fourth or fifth month of a female fetus' gestation and ends with menopause. A mature oocyte is called an ovum.
- Fertilization of the ovum occurs in the fallopian tube or oviduct. A fertilized ovum is called a zygote and becomes embedded in the uterine lining.
- The mammary glands function to produce and to release milk after childbirth.
- Hormones from the hypothalamus, anterior pituitary gland, and the gonads influence the female reproductive system.
- Female hormones are called estrogens.
- In women, gonadotropic hormones stimulate the formation of ova and the secretion of hormones from the sex organs.
- Menarche is the first menstrual period and marks the onset of puberty. Menstruation is the monthly flow of blood and other materials from the uterus. Menopause is when menstrual periods cease and the woman can no longer reproduce.
- The three phases of the ovarian cycle are the follicular phase, ovulation, and the luteal phase.
- The three phases of the uterine cycle are the proliferative phase, the secretory phase, and menstruation.

■ Teaching–Learning Strategies

CLASSROOM

1. Ask the students to define the following terms and abbreviations:

ERT	zygote
FSH	fimbriae
LH	ova
prolactin	mons pubis
oogenesis	vulva
oviducts	vagina
ovaries	menarche
clitoris	menopause
hymen	menstruation
endometrium	progesterone
labia	ovulation
mammary glands	uterus

Write the students' responses on the chalkboard or on an overhead transparency.

2. Show one or both of the following videotapes: *Reproduction in Humans* (27 minutes; available from Nimco, Inc., P.O. Box 9, 102 Highway 81 North, Calhoun, KY 42327) or *Human Reproductive Biology: Overcoming Infertility* (35 minutes; available from Films for the Humanities and Sciences, P.O. Box 2053, Princeton, NJ 08543-2053). After the videotape presentation, open the class for questions and discussion.

3. Invite a nurse who works with clients with gynecologic disorders to visit the class and present the role of the nurse in caring for female clients with reproductive disorders. After the presentation, open the class for questions and discussion.

CLINICAL

1. Demonstrate the various structures of the female reproductive system with charts or models. Ask students to identify major structures.

2. In the clinical setting, assign students to work with a nurse who is caring for female clients with reproductive disorders. Ask students to review the client's record and locate the physician's orders and laboratory or diagnostic findings related to the client's disorder. Ask the students to write their findings on a separate piece of paper.

Ask students to share their findings with the larger group.

3. Assign a small group of students to a diagnostic center or gynecologic center for female reproductive disorders or to an operating room setting where female reproductive surgery is performed. Ask students to share their observations with the larger group.

4. Role play a scenario and practice communication skills. Ask one student to volunteer to play the role of a female client who is infertile or going through menopause and ask the other student to play the role of the nurse. After the role-playing, ask students for comments and feedback.

5. Assign students to locate one article related to the reproductive system using the library or the Internet. Ask students to summarize their findings in a one- or two-page paper. Ask the students to share their findings with the larger group.

SUGGESTED RESOURCES: VIDEOTAPES

Approach to urinary incontinence in the elderly. (1988). [28 minutes]. (Available from Lippincott Williams & Wilkins, 530 Walnut Street, Philadelphia, PA 19106)

The art of breathing. [29 minutes]. (Available from Films for the Humanities and Sciences, P.O. Box 2053, Princeton, NJ 08543-2053)

Assessment set. (1997). [Set of three videotapes, 12–20 minutes each]. (Available from Lippincott Williams & Wilkins, 530 Walnut Street, Philadelphia, PA 19106)

Bates, B. (1995). *A visual guide to physical examination.* [Set of 12 videotapes, 17–25 minutes each]. (Available from Lippincott Williams & Wilkins, 530 Walnut Street, Philadelphia, PA 19106)

Causes of hearing loss. [18 minutes]. (Available from Films for the Humanities and Sciences, P.O. Box 2053, Princeton, NJ 08543-2053)

The heart: How it forms and functions. [25 minutes]. (Available from Films for the Humanities and Sciences, P.O. Box 2053, Princeton, NJ 08543-2053)

Insulin pump therapy. (1994). [20 minutes]. (Available from Lippincott Williams & Wilkins, 530 Walnut Street, Philadelphia, PA 19106)

Movements of joints of the body. [40 minutes]. (Available from Films for the Humanities and Sciences, P.O. Box 2053, Princeton, NJ 08543-2053)

Physical assessment. (1987). [Set of three videotapes, 20 minutes each]. (Available from Lippincott Williams & Wilkins, 530 Walnut Street, Philadelphia, PA 19106)

Prostate cancer. (1993). [7 minutes]. (Available from Lippincott Williams & Wilkins, 530 Walnut Street , Philadelphia, PA 19106)

Testicular examination. (1994). [5 minutes]. (Available from Lippincott Williams & Wilkins, 530 Walnut Street, Philadelphia, PA 19106)

Understanding ovarian cancer. (1994). [10 minutes].
(Available from Lippincott Williams & Wilkins, 530
Walnut Street, Philadelphia, PA 19106)

Women at midlife. [29 minutes]. (Available from Films for the
Humanities and Sciences, P.O. Box 2053, Princeton, NJ
08543-2053)

Your first pelvic exam. (1995). [8 minutes]. (Available from
Lippincott Williams & Wilkins, 530 Walnut Street,
Philadelphia, PA 19106)

ADDITIONAL RESOURCES

The Altruis Biomedical Network has two sites related
to the female reproductive system. The first site,
www.e-gynecologic.com, has links to the topics of
sexually transmitted diseases, hormones, anatomy of the
breast and uterus, puberty, birth control, osteoporosis,
pregnancy, and menopause. There also is a site on
hormones related to female reproduction: *www.e-
hormone.com*

AWHONN (Association of Women's Health, Obstetric, and
Neonatal Nurses; formerly NAACOG), website:
www.awhonn.org

Human Anatomy Online has a link to the topic of the female
reproductive system at
www.innerbody.com/htm/body.html.

CHAPTER 30

Basic Nutrition

LEARNING OBJECTIVES

1. Define nutrition and explain three functions of each of the six classes of major nutrients.

2. List the major dietary sources of carbohydrates and differentiate between monosaccharide, disaccharide, and polysaccharide.

3. Differentiate between saturated and unsaturated fatty acids. Explain cholesterol, LDL, and HDL.

4. Define amino acid. Differentiate between complete and incomplete proteins.

5. Explain the body's need for water and describe at least four functions of water.

6. List six major minerals and four trace minerals and state their functions.

7. Name the fat-soluble and water-soluble vitamins and list their main functions and food sources.

8. Identify the components of the Food Guide Pyramid and note the servings allotted for each compartment of the pyramid.

9. Discuss BMI, obesity, and malnutrition and how they relate to a healthy diet.

10. Identify at least three special nutritional considerations related to infancy, childhood, adolescence, early and middle adulthood, and the elderly.

NEW TERMINOLOGY

amino acid	monosaccharide
beriberi	nutrient
cholesterol	nutrient density
disaccharide	nutrition
essential nutrient	pellagra
glycogen	phytochemical
hydrogenated	polysaccharide
hyperglycemia	protein
hypoglycemia	rickets
lipid	saturated fat
macronutrients	scurvy
malnutrition	triglyceride
micronutrient	

KEY POINTS

- Essential nutrients (carbohydrates, fat, protein, water, minerals, and vitamins) provide energy, build and repair tissues, and regulate body processes.
- Kilocalories provide the body with needed energy.
- Carbohydrates provide energy, fiber, and sweetness. They spare protein.
- Fats supply energy, essential fatty acids, satiety, and flavor. They carry fat-soluble vitamins, protect organs, and regulate body temperature.
- Proteins repair and build body tissues, contribute to fluid and acid-base balance, form hormones and enzymes, and provide immune functions.
- Fat-soluble vitamins are vitamins A, D, E, and K; water-soluble vitamins are vitamin C and B complex.
- In healthy people, vitamins and minerals should not be supplemented in excess of the DRIs.
- The key concepts in diet planning are variety, balance, and moderation.
- Five of the 10 leading causes of death are related to an overconsumption of nutrients.
- No one food or food group can supply all necessary nutrients.
- Calcium, iron, and protein are important nutrients in the diets of infants, children, adolescents, and pregnant and lactating women.
- Nutritional needs and patterns of intake vary with age.

■ Teaching–Learning Strategies

CLASSROOM

1. Ask students to define the following terms and abbreviations:

ADA	GI
BMI	kcal
C (kilocalorie)	NE
CHO	RDA
DRI	REE
EAR	TE
ESADDI	UL

USDA   saturated fats
Fe   triglyceride
HDL   vitamin
IF   fiber
PCM   energy
PKU   enzyme
calcium   empty calories
iron   nutrient
potassium   nutrition
protein   overweight
magnesium   malnutrition
chloride   essential nutrients
obesity

Write the students' responses on the chalkboard or on an overhead transparency.

2. Begin the class with a discussion of basic nutrients. Ask students to group together in pairs. Assign each pair to a particular nutrient, mineral, or vitamin. Ask the students to determine the recommended dietary allowances and foods that are rich in the particular nutrient. Ask the pairs to share their findings with the larger group.

3. Ask a nutritionist to visit the class to discuss dietary needs across the lifespan. After the presentation, open the class for discussion, questions, and answers.

4. Conduct a discussion about general principles related to vitamins. Ask students to share their own experiences with taking vitamins.

5. Before class, ask students to keep a journal or diary with their food/fluid intake for 2 days. Ask the students to share their journals with another student in class and have each student evaluate the other student's dietary patterns. Ask each student to make suggestions or modifications as needed.

6. Before class, assign students to interview two individuals from different age groups about their dietary patterns. Ask students to share their findings with the larger group.

7. Assign a group of students to visit local supermarkets and a convenience store. Give the students a grocery list and ask them to compare the prices from each store. Ask the students to share their findings with the larger group. Conduct a discussion in class about the effects of poverty on dietary patterns and health and illness.

8. Compare and contrast obesity and malnutrition. Ask the students to identify how these conditions can affect one's state of health.

9. On an overhead transparency or the chalkboard, list the various lifespan categories. Ask the students to identify nutritional concerns and needs for each age group. List the students' responses.

CLINICAL

1. Take a small group of students to a healthcare facility. Ask the students to interview a staff member about the nutritional needs of the clients. Ask the students to share how the nurse is involved with nutritional planning and teaching of clients.

2. Invite a dietitian from a healthcare facility to meet with the students and discuss the various diets that must be planned for the clients. After the presentation, open the discussion for questions and answers.

3. Assign the students to a client who needs assistance with nutritional needs. Ask the students to assist the client during one meal. Ask the students to share their experiences and discuss the various diets of the clients.

4. Assign the students to observe a nurse or dietitian providing counseling to clients about their nutritional needs or special diets, such as a low-fat diet. Ask the students to share their experiences during clinical conference.

ADDITIONAL RESOURCES

American Diabetes Association, website: *www.diabetes.org*
American Dietetic Association, website: *www.eatright.org*
American Heart Association, website: *www.americanheart.org*

CHAPTER 31

Transcultural and Social Aspects of Nutrition

LEARNING OBJECTIVES

1. Explain the influence of region on food choices.

2. Identify common dietary practices of several ethnic groups.

3. Identify at least three dietary practices related to each of the following religions: Islam, Judaism, Mormon, and Roman Catholicism.

4. Name the four general types of vegetarian diets and identify what types of foods are eaten within each diet.

5. Describe how the lacto-ovo vegetarian can meet protein needs.

6. Relate the following factors to food choices: financial status, emotional state, social and physical factors, and ethnic heritage.

NEW TERMINOLOGY

kosher
soul food
tofu
tortillas
vegan
vegetarian
Yin–Yang

KEY POINTS

- Nurses play an important role in helping clients meet nutritional needs.
- To provide optimum care, understand the transcultural aspects of food and eating, and work within a person's cultural context to promote optimal nutrition.
- Ethnic and religious factors may plan an important part in food acceptance, especially during illness.
- Vegetarian diets are healthy and contain adequate protein if a wide variety of foods are eaten and calorie intake is sufficient. Pure vegans may need vitamin B_{12} and vitamin D supplements.

■ Teaching–Learning Strategies

CLASSROOM

1. During the class, review the concepts of ethnic influences on nutritional patterns and the relationship to health and illness.

2. Before class, on an overhead transparency, list various cultures (e.g., Hispanic) in one column. During class, ask the students to identify ethnic foods associated with the different cultures and potential health concerns. Write the students' responses on the transparency.

3. During class, ask students to share their own cultural preferences related to nutrition.

4. Before class, on an overhead transparency, list various religious groups (e.g., Roman Catholic) in one column. During class, ask students to identify foods associated with the different religious groups. Write the students' responses on the transparency.

5. Discuss ways to balance vegetarian diets.

6. Review other factors (e.g., loneliness) that can affect nutritional patterns. Ask students to share their own experiences related to social or economic factors and nutrition.

7. Ask students to prepare a food item related to their culture and bring it to class. During the class, ask students to share the origins of the food item and why it is important in their culture.

CLINICAL

1. In a clinical setting, assign students to a client whose culture is different from each student's culture. Ask students to interview the client

about their cultural nutrition preferences. Ask students to share their findings during clinical conference.

2. Ask a dietitian from a healthcare facility to visit the group and discuss ways that the healthcare facility attempts to incorporate cultural preferences of clients into the daily diets of the clients.

3. Ask students to visit an ethnic restaurant that is different from their own culture. Ask students to share their experiences with the group during clinical conference.

4. Before the clinical experience, ask students to design a vegetarian diet that is nutritionally adequate. Ask students to share their menu plans during clinical conference.

CHAPTER 32

Diet Therapy and Special Diets

LEARNING OBJECTIVES

1. Describe at least four roles of the nurse in providing nutritional support to a client in an acute care hospital, a long-term care facility, and a home care setting.

2. Identify the rationale for offering meal supplements, increasing fluids, or decreasing fluids.

3. Identify at least four reasons a client may need assistance with eating. State two nursing interventions for each type of circumstance.

4. Differentiate between the following types of diets: house diet, modified diet, and therapeutic diet.

5. State five methods of modifying diets in terms of nutrients, consistency, or energy.

6. Differentiate between a clear liquid and a full liquid diet. State the rationale and the limitations for the use of these diets.

7. Differentiate between a digestive soft and a mechanical soft diet. State the rationale and the limitations for the use of these diets.

8. Differentiate between a high residue and a low residue diet. State the rationale and the limitations for the use of these diets.

9. Explain three purposes of a carbohydrate-controlled diet.

10. Differentiate between the following diets: fat-controlled, low cholesterol, and limited saturated fats.

11. Explain the uses of low and high protein diets.

12. Identify the components of a mild, moderate, and severe sodium-restricted diet.

13. Demonstrate the procedure for the insertion of a nasogastric tube feeding.

14. Differentiate between TPN and PPN.

NEW TERMINOLOGY

anorexia	liquid diet
bland diet	low-residue diet
carbohydrate-controlled diet	modified diet
	polydipsia
dysphagia	soft diet
fat-controlled diet	stoma
hyperlipidemia	therapeutic diet
infusion	tube feeding
ketogenic diet	

KEY POINTS

- As a nurse, you play an important role in helping clients to meet their nutritional needs.
- Fluid is required to maintain homeostasis; too much plain water can lead to electrolyte imbalance.
- Documenting food and fluid intake is an important part of nursing care.
- Some individuals need special assistance to eat because of their age or a physical disorder.
- Modified diets are an important part of the treatment for many clients.
- The diet progression for "diet as tolerated" is clear liquid, full liquid, soft, regular (house).
- The carbohydrate-controlled or diabetic exchange lists for meal planning can be used for diabetic or weight-loss diets and in many other situations.
- Tube feeding is a commonly used means of providing nourishment and nutritional support.

■ Teaching–Learning Strategies

CLASSROOM

1. Ask the students to define the following terms and abbreviations:

FF	Stat
G tube	TPN
J tube	I & O
Na	IV
NPO	anorexia
PEG	bulimia

infusion   stoma
dysphagia   edema
polydipsia   supplement
hyperlipidemia total parenteral nutrition

Write the students' responses on the chalkboard or on an overhead transparency.

2. Review the suggested strategies for preparing clients for meals and serving food. Ask students why it is important to prepare clients for mealtimes.

3. Before class, on 3 × 5 index cards, write various modified diets (e.g., sodium restricted, calorie restricted). During class, divide the class into groups of two. Give each pair an index card. Ask the students to plan a menu for a 24-hour period to meet the dietary guidelines for each diet. Ask the students to share their plans with the larger group. Ask students to identify nutrients that may be lacking in these diets.

4. During the class, ask the students to identify risk factors related to food and nutrient intake. On an overhead transparency, list the students' responses.

5. Bring several nonperishable food items to the class, such as canned vegetables, meats, soup, noodles, and beans. Distribute the items in class and ask students to read the various labels that identify the products' contents. Ask students to share their observations with the larger class.

CLINICAL

1. In the clinical laboratory, ask the students to view the videotape *Enteral Feeding 2E* (20 minutes; available from Lippincott Williams & Wilkins, 530 Walnut Street, Philadelphia, PA 19106). After the videotape presentation, open the class for questions and discussion.

2. In the clinical laboratory, provide examples of various enteral feeding supplies and equipment. Ask the students to practice intermittent (bolus) or continuous feedings using the equipment. Answer questions as needed. After the practice

session, ask the students to document in the record/chart of a fictitious client.

3. Bring various types of foods/fluids to the clinical laboratory to demonstrate clear liquid, full liquid, soft, and low-residue dietary products. Have pairs of students practice planning various diets. Ask the students to role play feeding various clients who need assistance with feeding, such as those who are visually impaired, have difficulty with swallowing, or lack an appetite. Ask the students to share their feelings after the role-playing experience.

4. In the clinical setting, assign each student to a client who needs assistance with feeding or nutrition. If possible, assign several students to clients who are receiving enteral feedings. Ask each student to prepare the client for meals, serve the food tray, and provide needed assistance. After the mealtime, ask the students to document in the client's record.

SUGGESTED RESOURCES: VIDEOTAPES

Cholesterol control: An eater's guide. [30 minutes]. (Available from Lippincott Williams & Wilkins, 530 Walnut Street, Philadelphia, PA 19106)
Food-borne illnesses and their prevention. [35 minutes]. (Available from Films for the Humanities and Sciences, P.O. Box 2053, Princeton, NJ 08543-2053, 800-257-5126)
Good nutrition for people with HIV/AIDS. [6 minutes]. (Available from Lippincott Williams & Wilkins, 530 Walnut Street, Philadelphia, PA 19106)
The nurse's guide to enteral feeding tubes. [32 minutes]. (Available from Insight Media, P.O. Box 621, New York, NY 10024)
Nutrition and cancer. [21 minutes]. (Available from Films for the Humanities and Sciences, P.O. Box 2053, Princeton, NJ 08543-2053; 800-257-5126.)
Nutritional assessment of the elderly. (1988). [28 minutes]. (Available from Lippincott Williams & Wilkins, 530 Walnut Street, Philadelphia, PA 19106)
Osteoporosis: Progress and prevention. [24 minutes]. (Available from Films for the Humanities and Sciences, P.O. Box 2053, Princeton, NJ 08543-2053; 800-257-5126)
Our overweight kids. (1998). [28 minutes]. (Available from Aquarius Health Care Videos, P.O. Box 1159, Sherborn, MA 01770)
Understanding eating disorders. (1996). [26 minutes]. (Available from Aquarius Health Care Videos, P.O. Box 1159, Sherborn, MA 01770)

CHAPTER 33

Introduction to the Nursing Process

LEARNING OBJECTIVES

1. Define the new terminology
2. Explain the use of critical thinking to solve problems.
3. Discuss the relationship between critical thinking and problem solving.
4. Explain the use of the nursing process in nursing practice.
5. Describe the nurse's actions during each step of the nursing process.
6. Compare the seven steps of scientific problem solving with the correlated steps of the nursing process.

NEW TERMINOLOGY

client oriented	nursing process
critical thinking	scientific problem solving
nursing care plans	trial and error

KEY POINTS

- Scientists have used scientific problem solving for many years to systematize their research.
- Critical thinking is an important nursing strategy for problem solving.
- The nursing process is a framework of scientific problem solving combined with critical thinking skills.
- The nursing process provides individualized care that is accountable.
- Steps in the nursing process include assessment, nursing diagnosis, planning, implementation, and evaluation.
- The nursing process can be used to identify not only the client's actual problems, but also potential problems.
- The client and the family are involved in developing the nursing care plan.

■ Teaching–Learning Strategies

CLASSROOM

1. Display a chart outlining the differences between the trial and error and scientific problem solving methods of problem solving. Ask the students to verbalize their understanding of these methods and to compare them to the nursing process.

2. Guide the students to develop a practical definition of a critical thinker. Lead a discussion to allow each student to evaluate his or her own critical thinking skills.

3. Divide students into five groups and appoint a spokesperson and recorder. Ask each group to define and identify strategies necessary to implement each step of the nursing process.

CLINICAL

1. Assign students to observe and confer with nurses at work in an acute care facility. Have students identify the stage of the nursing process in which the nurses are functioning. Allow students to share their findings in postconference.

2. Instruct students to observe and confer with nurses at work in a long-term care facility. Have students identify the stage of the nursing process at which the nurses are functioning. Allow students to share their experiences in the postconference.

3. Allow students to discuss specific actions carried out by the staff during the nursing process.

SUGGESTED RESOURCES: WEBSITES

home.hiwaay.net/~theholt1/NURS1100/class1.htm
www2.nau.edu/~erw/nur301/practice/process/lesson.html

CHAPTER 34

Nursing Assessment

LEARNING OBJECTIVES

1. Define the key terms.

2. Discuss the steps in nursing assessment.

3. Differentiate between subjective and objective data.

4. Explain methods of data collection.

5. Identify techniques used in the health interview.

6. Discuss the process of data analysis to determine client problems.

NEW TERMINOLOGY

data analysis
health interview
nursing assessment
nursing history
objective data
observation
subjective data

Acronyms

ADL, activities of daily living
CC, chief complaint
JCAHO, Joint Commission on Accreditation of Healthcare Organizations

KEY POINTS

- Nursing assessment is the systematic gathering of data about the client.
- Assessment uses observation (the senses), the interview, and the physical examination.
- Data collected include objective data (factual, measurable, what you can observe) and subjective (what the client tells you, the client's opinions and feelings).

- Data analysis requires recognizing patterns or clusters, identifying strengths and problems, and reaching conclusions.

■ Teaching–Learning Strategies

CLASSROOM

1. Display the steps of the nursing process on the chalkboard or an overhead transparency. Present the nursing process as the framework for collecting pertinent client data.

2. Obtain standard nursing assessment forms from various healthcare facilities. Allow students to review these forms. Entertain questions.

3. Present and distribute specific forms for documenting nursing process data for this course.

CLINICAL

1. Assign students to work in pairs to review charts or assessment forms on an assigned clinical unit.

2. Have students observe nursing assessment data on the chart and determine if conclusions can be made about the client based on the data documented.

3. Have students ask the following questions about the client based on the data documented: Do the data give a complete picture of the client? How could the data be more complete?

CHAPTER 35

Diagnosis and Planning

LEARNING OBJECTIVES

1. Define the key terms.

2. Differentiate between nursing diagnosis and medical diagnosis.

3. State the purposes of nursing diagnosis.

4. Explain the components of nursing diagnosis.

5. List the steps in planning client care, and describe how nurses carry out these steps.

6. Describe the purpose and format of the nursing care plan.

NEW TERMINOLOGY

collaborative problem
expected outcome
Kardex
long-term objective
medical diagnosis
nursing care plan
nursing diagnosis
planning
prognosis
short-term objective

KEY POINTS

- Nursing diagnosis is a statement about the client's actual or potential health concerns that can be managed through independent nursing interventions.
- A medical diagnosis is concerned with the disease process. A nursing diagnosis is concerned with the person and how the disease affects his or her functioning.
- Nursing diagnosis helps identify nursing priorities and goals to maintain quality and continuity of care.
- Nursing diagnosis is stated in terms of a problem (statement approved by NANDA), its etiology, and signs and symptoms.
- After establishing nursing diagnoses, the planning nursing care begins. Priorities, expected outcomes, and nursing interventions are selected; a nursing care plan is written.

■ Teaching–Learning Strategies

CLASSROOM

1. On an overhead transparency or chalkboard, outline the differences between the medical and nursing diagnosis.

2. Ask students to provide the three components of the nursing diagnosis.

3. Allow students to verbalize the role of the practical nurse in developing and implementing the nursing diagnosis.

4. Display examples of nursing diagnostic statements on an overhead transparency. Allow students to identify the three parts to the diagnosis and to practice identifying diagnostic statements and interventions.

5. Lead a discussion focusing on the purpose of developing "client-focused" expected outcomes.

CLINICAL

1. Divide the class in pairs to assist a nurse at work on a unit. Instruct them to concentrate their attention on the diagnosing and planning aspects of the nursing process. Inform the staff of the student's focus and encourage the staff to verbalize their decision-making process. Allow students to share their experiences in postconference.

2. Obtain care plan forms from several healthcare facilities and allow the students to observe the diversity of these care plans.

3. Allow two students to interview a client using the standard documentation forms to begin to collect client data necessary to develop the nursing diagnosis and to plan care.

CHAPTER 36

Implementing and Evaluating Care

LEARNING OBJECTIVES

1. Define the key terms.

2. List the major steps in carrying out nursing interventions (implementation).

3. Compare and contrast intellectual (cognitive), interpersonal (affective), and technical (psychomotor) skills and describe how they apply to nursing.

4. List the steps in evaluating nursing care and describe how they might be accomplished.

5. Describe at least three means used for evaluating client care.

6. Define quality assurance, chart audit, and nursing peer review.

7. Describe discharge planning.

NEW TERMINOLOGY

accountability	independent actions
case management	intellectual skills
case manager	interdependent actions
chart audit	interpersonal skills
clinical care path	nursing peer review
dependent actions	quality assurance
discharge planning	technical skills
evaluation	variance
implementation	

KEY POINTS

- Implementation involves dependent, interdependent, and independent actions.
- Nurses use intellectual, interpersonal, and technical skills to implement care plans.
- During implementation, nurses collect additional data and communicate information with other members of the healthcare team.

- Some facilities use a system of managed care to increase cost effectiveness while maintaining quality care.
- Evaluate client responses and revise the nursing care plan as needed.
- Quality assurance programs use nursing care plans and other documentation to evaluate quality of care.
- Discharge planning and future planning are based on nursing care plans.

■ Teaching–Learning Strategies

CLASSROOM

1. As students enter the classroom, have the definition of implementation projected on an overhead transparency.

2. Lead a brief discussion about the types of nursing actions and skills required in the implementation and evaluation stages of the nursing process.

3. Divide the class into two groups. Instruct each group to develop examples of the strategies needed to implement the above steps of the nursing process.

4. Discuss managed healthcare delivery systems. Ask students to identify how managed care impinges on planning methods of the nurse.

5. On an overhead transparency, outline the components of quality assurance and discharge planning. Lead a discussion about these.

6. Obtain critical pathway forms and protocol forms from an acute healthcare facility for students to review.

CLINICAL

1. Assign students in pairs to one client in an acute healthcare facility.

2. Lead students in a chart review to observe the documentation of nursing care, critical/care pathway forms, and nursing protocol forms.

3. Instruct students to complete a nursing assessment at the level of their understanding using the concepts and documentation forms given them.

CHAPTER 37

Documenting and Reporting

LEARNING OBJECTIVES

1. State at least three reasons for maintaining a health record.

2. Explain the differences between manual and electronic documentation.

3. List four categories of information included in the health record.

4. Describe various formats for organizing nursing progress notes.

5. State generally accepted guidelines for documentation.

6. Give descriptive terminology for client signs and symptoms when documenting client care.

7. Identify common abbreviations when documenting client care.

8. State the correct way to record a documentation error, and differentiate a documentation error from a client care error.

9. Explain how and when to report to other nursing staff.

NEW TERMINOLOGY

change-of-shift reporting
confidentiality
flow sheet
health record
medical information system
medication administration record
minimum data set
progress note
walking rounds

KEY POINTS

- The primary purposes of the health record are to facilitate communication among caregivers, to provide evidence of accountability, and to facilitate health research and education. Both manual and electronic records serve these purposes.

- Electronic records use medical information systems to enter, store, process, and retrieve client data.
- Assessment documents record all client information.
- Minimum data sets and resident assessment protocols guide nurses to develop individualized care plans, especially in long-term and home care.
- Plans for treatment of the client include the physician's orders and the nursing care plan.
- Progress records describe the treatment and responses of the client.
- Healthcare facilities use various formats to organize nursing progress notes in the health record.
- Plans for the continuity of care include teaching plans, transfer notes, and discharge summaries.
- Accurate and complete documentation ensures effective communication and accountability.
- Confidentiality is a client's right to privacy that healthcare personnel safeguard in both documentation and reporting.
- Reporting is an oral method of communication that is timely, precise, and accurate.

■ Teaching–Learning Strategies

CLASSROOM

1. On an overhead transparency, outline the contents of the health record and its purpose.

2. Obtain examples of the manual (paper) health record for students to peruse.

3. Allow students to share their thoughts and feelings when information about them had to be recorded on a health record.

4. Distribute written scenarios of a client assessment. Divide students into groups and allow them to decide what information should be reported.

5. Assign students to present a scenario of "reporting off" at the end of a shift to another nurse regarding the status of her clients.

6. Allow students to quiz each other regarding common abbreviations for observations used in the health record.

7. Show the videotape *Documenting Nursing Practice* (1993; 28 minutes; available from Insight Media, #888, P.O. Box 621, New York, NY 10024).

CLINICAL

1. Take students to a clinical unit to observe common abbreviations used in documentation.

2. Ask the students to make note of how many abbreviations they can recall without using class notes? Ask how many parts of the health record they can identify?

3. Instruct students to be prepared to answer the following questions:

   • What type of nursing note format is used by the staff?
   • Are the nursing notes manually or electronically documented? Or both?

   Allow students to present their findings in clinical conference.

SUGGESTED RESOURCES

Alfaro-LeFevre, R. (1998). *Applying nursing process: A step-by-step approach* (4th ed.). Philadelphia: Lippincott Williams & Wilkins.

Collier, I. C., et al. (1996). *Writing nursing diagnosis: A critical thinking approach*. St. Louis: Mosby.

Gulanick, M., et al. (Eds.). (1997). *Nursing care plans: Nursing diagnosis and intervention*. St. Louis: Mosby.

Hill, S. S., & Howlett, H. A. (1997). *Success in practical nursing: Personal and vocational issues*. Philadelphia: Saunders.

Kneafsey, R. (1998). Success in practical nursing: Personal and vocational issues. *Journal of Advanced Nursing, 27*(5), 1098.

Sparks, S. M., & Taylor, C. M. (1998). *Nursing diagnosis reference manual*. Springhouse, PA: Springhouse.

CHAPTER 38

The Healthcare Facility Environment

LEARNING OBJECTIVES

1. List and describe components included in the basic client unit.

2. Compare and contrast the basic client unit in the hospital, long-term care, and home care settings.

3. Discuss the relationship between housekeeping procedures and client safety.

4. Summarize the guidelines for all nursing procedures.

5. Describe at least four direct client care departments in hospitals.

6. Describe the functions of at least four hospital support departments.

KEY TERMS

autopsy	ophthalmology
client unit	otoscope
commode	pathologist
intercom	pediatric
morgue	physical therapy
neurodiagnostic	protocol
nuclear medicine	rationale
nursing unit	research laboratory
obstetrics	respiratory therapy
occupational therapy	telecommunications
operating room	telehealth

KEY POINTS

- The needs of clients include the basic needs of all human beings plus special needs connected with illness or injury.
- The client unit is the area in which you deliver most nursing care.
- The client care unit in the hospital, extended care facility, and home is designed to meet healthcare needs.
- A clean and orderly unit helps to prevent accidents and infections.
- Certain guidelines are common for all nursing procedures. Some procedures are grouped according to time of day.
- Healthcare facilities offer a wide variety of services and often are staffed with personnel who have special training. Direct client care departments, specialized client care departments, and support services are found within many facilities.
- Many services provided in the hospital also are provided in extended care facilities, clinics, and the home.

■ Teaching–Learning Strategies

CLASSROOM

1. Ask students to define the following terms:

autopsies	physical therapy
research laboratory	nuclear medicine
client unit	telecommunications
commode	occupational therapy
dietary department	rehabilitation unit
Mayo stand	dialysis unit
morgue	hospice
pathologist	

   Write the students' responses on the chalkboard or on an overhead transparency.

2. Ask students to identify the components of the basic client unit. Write the students' responses on the chalkboard or on an overhead transparency.

3. Review general guidelines for performing nursing procedures. Ask students to share personal experiences about hospitalization either of themselves or a family member.

4. Divide the class into four groups. Assign each group a specific time of day for nursing care (e.g., early morning care). Ask each group to identify the types of activities that are performed during this time period. Write the students' responses on the chalkboard or on an overhead transparency.

5. On an overhead transparency or the chalkboard write in four columns: diagnostic and treatment departments, direct client care departments, specialized client care departments, and support services. Ask the students to identify various services under each category. Write the responses on the chalkboard or on an overhead transparency.

6. Invite a nurse who is employed in a home health agency to visit the class and discuss how home care differs from hospital care. After the presentation, open the class for questions and discussion.

CLINICAL

1. While students are assigned to a hospital unit, ask each student to review the hospital's policy and procedure manuals. Ask students to look up one specific procedure and report the procedure during clinical conference.

2. Assign a small group of students to a nurse employed in a home health or rehabilitation setting. After the experience, ask the students to share their observations during clinical conference.

3. Assign a small group of students to an outpatient setting. Ask the students to assist a nurse in the clinic for the clinical day. Ask students to share their experiences during clinical conference.

4. Assign students in pairs to visit other units (e.g., occupational therapy) within the hospital setting. Ask students to write a one- to two-page report on their observations and make a verbal report during clinical conference.

CHAPTER 39

Emergency Preparedness

LEARNING OBJECTIVES

1. List at least 10 nursing measures that help to prevent accidents in the healthcare facility.

2. Identify five potentially hazardous materials.

3. Describe the use of a material safety data sheet (MSDS).

4. Describe at least five safety tips to consider when using and storing hazardous substances.

5. Explain the use of the emergency signal.

6. Identify alternate methods of communication when a disruption occurs in telephone service.

7. List at least five things to consider when developing a personal emergency preparedness plan.

8. Discuss the difference between an internal and external disaster.

9. Describe actions to take when a bomb threat occurs.

10. Define triage.

11. List three things to consider when evacuation from a facility or a client's home is necessary.

12. Explain the acronym RACE and its relation to the fire plan.

13. List four classes of fire extinguishers and their uses.

NEW TERMINOLOGY

command center
disaster medical assistance team
employee right-to-know laws
external disaster
internal disaster
simple triage and rapid treatment
triage

KEY POINTS

- The safety committee functions in evaluating accidents that have occurred and in planning to prevent future occurrences.
- Nurses not only must prevent accidents but also must know what to do if an accident occurs.
- Staff members must be able to identify potentially hazardous substances and describe what to do if exposed to them.
- A personal emergency preparedness plan will help you to cope with the disruption caused by a disaster and focus on caring for clients.
- A facility's disaster plan is set up to deal with internal and external emergencies.
- Every staff member in a healthcare facility or community setting must be knowledgeable about fire safety.

■ Teaching–Learning Strategies

CLASSROOM

1. Ask students to define the following terms:

   command center
   triage
   external disaster
   employee right-to-know laws
   hazardous substances
   emergency resuscitation
   internal disaster
   RACE

   Write the students' responses on the chalkboard or on an overhead transparency.

2. Ask students to identify methods for preventing accidents, such as falls. Write the students' responses on the chalkboard or on an overhead transparency.

3. Briefly discuss guidelines for fire prevention. Ask the students to identify a plan for evacuation during a fire in a hospital or home setting. Write the students' responses on the chalkboard or on an overhead transparency.

4. Ask a nurse who is employed in a hospital and who is on the emergency response team to visit the class and discuss internal and external disaster preparedness. After the presentation, open the class for questions and discussion. Ask students to identify their own personal preparedness procedures.

CLINICAL

1. While in a hospital setting, ask students to review the hospital's policy and procedure manual for plans for internal and external disasters. Ask students to share their findings during clinical conference.

2. Ask students to assess their house or apartment for potential fire or other safety hazards. Ask students to write a one- to two-page plan for correcting these hazards and share their plans during clinical conference.

3. Assign a small group of students to make home visits with a home health nurse. Ask students to observe any potential safety hazards in the client's setting. Ask students to share their observations during clinical conference.

4. Assign students in pairs to locate hazardous chemicals or gases on the clinical unit. Ask students to locate fire extinguishers for their unit and share their findings during clinical conference.

5. Assign a pair of students to a hospital emergency room. Ask students to interview a nurse who has experienced an internal or an external disaster. Ask students to share their findings during clinical conference.

WEB RESOURCE

Professional Safeguard Resources, website: *www.psrcorp.com*

CHAPTER 40

Microbiology and Defense Against Disease

LEARNING OBJECTIVES

1. Explain what microorganisms are and why an understanding of them is vital for all healthcare workers.

2. Define the term *pathogen*.

3. Name and describe the essential factors that influence microbial growth.

4. Describe how culture and sensitivity reports and staining aid in the treatment of infectious diseases.

5. Identify the basic characteristics of the five main types of microorganisms.

6. Describe the way in which bacteria are classified.

7. Discuss ways to prevent the development of drug-resistant bacteria.

8. Explain three basic ways in which infectious diseases are transmitted to people.

9. Name the components of the chain of infection.

10. Suggest ways in which to stop the spread of infection at each point in the chain.

11. Describe the effect of toxins on the body.

12. Describe factors that help determine if a pathogen will cause disease.

NEW TERMINOLOGY

aerobe	mycosis
anaerobe	opportunistic
bacillus	parasite
bacteria	pathogen
bacteriology	prodromal
communicable	reservoir
contagious	sensitivity
culture	spirillum
endemic	spore
endotoxin	sterile
epidemic	suppurative
etiology	toxin
exotoxin	vector
flagellum	virulence
incubation period	virus
microorganisms	

KEY POINTS

- Some microorganisms are beneficial in nature. Others, called pathogens, cause disease in human beings.
- All microorganisms, except viruses, engage in the same life functions as do other plant and animal cells. Their reproduction and infectious spread in human beings depend on the right set of environmental conditions.
- Culture and sensitivity reports and staining identify microorganisms and appropriate treatment for them.

- Microorganisms are classified by their physical and biologic characteristics into basic groups, each with distinguishing means of reproducing and (if they are pathogens) of infecting people.
- With the number of drug-resistant and multidrug-resistant bacteria increasing, prudent use of antibiotics is essential.
- Viruses cause disease by taking over the host cell's metabolism and genetic material and by reproducing in extremely large numbers.
- Most common microbial diseases are communicable and are spread within the population by direct or indirect contact; contaminated air, water, or food; or through vectors.
- Healthcare professionals who practice antiseptic techniques and Standard Precautions can break the chain of infection.
- Infections follow a progressive course. Many factors contribute to the microorganism's ability to result in disease.

■ Teaching–Learning Strategies

CLASSROOM

1. Ask students to define the following terms:

bacteria	vector
communicable	portal of entry
microorganism	opportunistic
pathogen	endemic
sterile	epidemic
contagious	toxin
mycosis	virulence
suppurative	incubation period
endotoxin	parasite
host	virus

Write the students' responses on the chalkboard or on an overhead transparency.

2. Invite a microbiologist to visit the class and discuss the topic of microorganisms and disease.

After the presentation, open the class for questions and discussion.

3. Ask students to share their personal experiences with various diseases, such as chickenpox, colds, or flu. Ask students to identify possible portals of entry, vector, and vehicle of transmission.

4. Assign students to grow mold at home or bring some mold on food to class for the students to observe. Show drawings or photographs of various bacteria during the class. Ask students to discuss the role of the nurse in prevention of disease transmission.

CLINICAL

1. Assign a small group of students to visit the laboratory of a hospital. Ask students to observe and report their observations to the group during clinical conference.

2. Ask students to review the policy or procedure manual and locate items related to prevention of disease transmission. Ask students to share their findings during clinical conference.

3. While on the clinical unit, ask students to observe the various personnel to determine how disease transmission is prevented. Ask the students to share their observations during clinical conference.

4. Assign students in pairs to design a poster on the topic of disease prevention. Ask students to share their posters during clinical conference.

5. Assign students in pairs a particular disease. Ask students to research the Internet to determine the incidence of the disease in the local community. Ask students to share their findings during clinical conference.

CHAPTER 41

Medical Asepsis

LEARNING OBJECTIVES

1. Explain what is meant by a *nosocomial infection*.

2. Identify at least three factors that predispose clients to nosocomial infections.

3. Target ways that nurses can avoid contracting and spreading nosocomial infections.

4. Define medical asepsis.

5. Describe the elements of medical asepsis.

6. Perform skills in handwashing.

7. Demonstrate the use of appropriate barrier techniques.

8. Explain how antimicrobial agents and environmental controls contribute to medical asepsis.

9. Identify reasons for teaching asepsis to clients and families.

NEW TERMINOLOGY

antimicrobial agent	invasive
asepsis	medical asepsis
bacteremia	nosocomial infection
endogenous	personal protective
exogenous	equipment

KEY POINTS

- Nosocomial infections are acquired in healthcare facilities.
- Clients are more susceptible to infections in healthcare facilities because their resistance to disease often is lowered, and facilities house many pathogens.
- Medical asepsis helps lower the number of microorganisms in the environment and prevents and reduces their transmission.
- Handwashing is the single most important skill in the prevention of disease spread.

- Commonly used protective barriers include gloves, eye protection, gowns, and masks.
- Keeping a clean and controlled environment is essential to maintaining medical asepsis.
- Antimicrobial agents limit and destroy pathogens. Commonly used examples include antiseptics and disinfectants.
- Following proper methods of leaving a client's room; the use of mask, gowns, and gloves; and terminal disinfection help prevent infections.
- Teaching aseptic practices to clients, families, and visitors is essential for protection against disease, particularly because clients often leave the healthcare facility while they are still ill.

■ Teaching–Learning Strategies

CLASSROOM

1. Ask students to define the following terms:

antimicrobial agents	invasive
exogenous	bacteremia
personal protective	nosocomial infections
equipment	barrier
asepsis	endogenous
sterilization	contaminated

Write the students' responses on the chalkboard or on an overhead transparency.

2. During the class, show the videotape *Washing Hands* (1993; 20 minutes; available from Insight Media, P.O. Box 621, New York, NY 10024). After the videotape presentation, open the class for questions and discussion.

3. During the class, show the videotape *Medical Asepsis and Infection Prevention* (1993; 15 minutes; available from Nimco, Inc., P.O. Box 9, 102 Highway 81 North, Calhoun, KY 42327). After the videotape presentation, open the class for questions and discussion.

4. Bring a variety of soaps and disinfecting agents from home to the classroom. Ask students to compare and contrast the various agents. Write the students' observations on the chalkboard or on an overhead transparency.

5. Briefly discuss guidelines for preventing infections. Ask students to differentiate endogenous and exogenous microorganisms. Write the students' observations on the chalkboard or on an overhead transparency.

CLINICAL

1. Assign students to practice handwashing and scrubbing for an operative procedure either in the learning laboratory or the clinical setting. During clinical conference, ask students to discuss why handwashing is so important in client care.

2. Assign a pair of students to observe individuals in a public restroom for a short period of time. Ask students to share their findings related to the number of individuals who entered the restroom compared to the number of individuals who washed their hands.

3. In the learning laboratory, have students practice barrier techniques for clients in isolation or for the operating room. Ask students to share their feelings about wearing protective barrier equipment.

4. Assign one or two students to care for a client who is in isolation. Ask students to share their experiences during clinical conference.

ADDITIONAL RESOURCES

Centers for Disease Control and Prevention, website: *www.cdc.gov*
Occupational Safety and Health Administration, website: *www.osha.gov*

CHAPTER 42

Infection Control

LEARNING OBJECTIVES

1. Explain the relationship between standard and transmission-based precautions and infection control.

2. Discuss the purpose, use, and components of Standard Precautions.

3. Explain the purpose, use, and components of transmission-based precautions.

4. Identify how to follow specific airborne, droplet, and contact precautions.

5. Describe how to set up a client's room for isolation and appropriate barrier techniques.

6. Demonstrate precautions to take during medication administration, vital sign monitoring, and transport of a client who is potentially infectious.

7. Explain what is meant by protective (neutropenic/reverse) isolation.

8. Identify the role of the infection control committee.

NEW TERMINOLOGY

airborne precautions
colonization
contact precautions
droplet precautions
isolation

neutropenic isolation
protective isolation
Standard Precautions
transmission-based
  precautions

KEY POINTS

- Infection is best controlled by prevention—breaking the links in the chain of infection.
- The Joint Commission on the Accreditation of Healthcare Organizations (JCAHO) requires every healthcare facility it accredits to have an infection control plan.
- Standard Precautions consider that every client's blood and body fluids are potentially infectious; thus, Standard Precautions are used in the care of all clients.

- Transmission-based precautions are designed to prevent the spread of specific infections. They include airborne, droplet, and contact precautions. The specific type of transmission-based precautions for a particular client is used in conjunction with Standard Precautions.
- Barrier techniques prevent microorganisms from leaving a client's room.
- Special filtered respirator masks are often required when caring for a client with known or suspected tuberculosis.
- Before entering a client's room, assess to determine needed PPE and other equipment needed.
- Isolation often is frightening and misunderstood by clients and families.
- Isolation procedures vary among healthcare facilities. Know your facility's specific procedures.
- Protective isolation prevents organisms from coming into contact with clients.
- One duty of an infection control committee is to monitor and evaluate infections in clients and in staff who are exposed.

■Teaching–Learning Strategies

CLASSROOM

1. Ask students to define the following terms or give examples:

   Standard Precautions
   transmission-based precautions
   droplet precautions
   contact precautions
   isolation
   reverse isolation

2. Ask students to identify a basis outline of Standard Precautions. Write the students' responses on the chalkboard or on an overhead transparency. Briefly discuss transmission-based precautions.

3. Ask students to describe how they would set up an isolation room in a hospital setting. Write the students' responses on the chalkboard or on an overhead transparency.

4. Briefly discuss the care of a dead body using Standard Precautions. Ask students to identify various precautions that need to be taken.

5. Briefly review neutropenic or reverse isolation procedures. Ask the students to identify types of situations where reverse isolation would be necessary. Write the students' responses on the chalkboard or on an overhead transparency.

CLINICAL

1. In the learning laboratory, divide the students into groups of two. Ask each pair to role play a situation whereby one of the students is the client in isolation and the other is the nurse. Have the students practice various procedures for clients in isolation.

2. Arrange for a pair of students to attend an institution's infection control committee meeting.

Ask the students to share their experiences during clinical conference.

3. Ask students to do Internet or library research to identify causes of infection in healthcare settings. Ask the students what procedures they can use to help reduce the incidence of infection in hospital settings.

4. Assign one or two students to work with a nurse on a hospital unit who is caring for a client in isolation. Ask the students to interview the nurse or the client about nursing care for such clients.

5. Arrange for a pair of students to observe in an operating room that is using controlled ventilation. Ask the students to share their experiences with the larger group.

WEB RESOURCES

The Centers for Disease Control and Prevention, website: *www.cdc.gov*
The Occupational Safety and Health Administration, website: *www.osha.gov*
The World Health Organization workshop regarding the containment of antimicrobial resistance, website: *http://www.who.int/m/topics/antimicrobial-resistant_bacterial_infections/en/index.html*

CHAPTER 43

Emergency Care and First Aid

LEARNING OBJECTIVES

1. Discuss the importance of assessing the safety of an emergency scene.

2. Describe the medical identification tag and its purpose.

3. Describe, in order, the steps for assessing an ill or injured person in an emergency.

4. Identify early, common, and progressive signs of shock.

5. Describe at least five common types of shock, including hypovolemic shock, identifying nursing actions in emergency-induced shock.

6. Define sudden death.

7. Differentiate between clinical and biologic death.

8. State and demonstrate the procedure for calling a code in your healthcare facility or agency.

9. Describe emergency actions for chest, neck, back, and head injuries.

10. In the lab, demonstrate emergency actions for a puncture wound of the chest.

11. Describe at least three signs of increasing intracranial pressure.

12. Explain symptoms and first aid for injuries caused by exposure to cold, including frostbite and hypothermia.

13. Describe symptoms and immediate first aid for heat-related illnesses and injuries, including heat exhaustion and severe burns.

14. List at least three signs of inhalation injury after a fire.

15. Discuss first aid for musculoskeletal injuries, including a fracture, demonstrating the ability to safely splint an ulnar or radial fracture using common household materials.

16. Describe the immediate actions of a rescuer in suspected heart attack.

17. Describe emergency care for at least three different types of hemorrhage.

18. Define the term *anaphylaxis* and describe causes, symptoms, and treatment of anaphylaxis.

19. Identify at least three precautions to take when dealing with hazardous materials.

20. List at least five immediate actions to take when a person is suspected of being poisoned.

21. Define the term *triage* and describe how it applies to emergency care.

22. List at least four factors that identify a psychiatric emergency or the potential for suicide.

NEW TERMINOLOGY

ambu bag	hypothermia
anaphylaxis	intrusion (injury)
antidote	intubation
avulsion (injury)	mediastinal shift
bandage	near drowning
biologic death	pneumothorax
café coronary	poison
caustic	rabies
clinical death	shock
code	splint
debride	sprain
dislocation	strain
emetic	stridor
epistaxis	sudden death
extrication	syncope
fracture frostbite	thrombolytic
gastric lavage	tourniquet
heat cramps	toxin
heat exhaustion	trauma
heat stroke	triage
hemorrhage	wind chill factor

KEY POINTS

- Nurses are with clients much of the time in the healthcare facility. Thus, they may be in the position to recognize and alert the appropriate staff to deal with cardiopulmonary arrest and other emergencies.
- Nurses must use Standard Precautions (to whatever extent possible) when administering first aid.
- In emergencies, nurses and nursing students function only at their level of first aid training. Quick evaluation of the scene and planning for action are crucial.
- Calling 911 will summon the EMS system in almost all areas of the United States and Canada. The nurse must know how to summon assistance in an emergency.
- When assessing an emergency, the most important consideration is to make sure the person is breathing and that his or her heart is beating.
- Be sure to treat the injured person for shock.
- Do not move an injured person unless the situation is dangerous. Take precautions to prevent additional injury.
- All healthcare workers, including nurses, should know how to perform CPR in an emergency. Maintain current CPR certification.
- The nurse may be called on to provide first aid assistance in a community. Each nurse has the responsibility to be knowledgeable in basic first aid techniques.
- Chest injuries can result in inadequate air exchange and be immediately life threatening. Ensure the chest wall is intact. Plug any open wound of the chest. Do not remove any penetrating objects.
- Be aware of the possibility of injury from excessive heat or cold. Take prompt action in life-threatening situations.
- A person who is having a heart attack often is in denial. The EMS personnel may need to be very persuasive to get the victim to appropriate medical care.

■ Teaching–Learning Strategies

CLASSROOM

1. Ask the students to define the following terms or abbreviations:

CPR	sudden infant death
heat cramps	syndrome
shock	emetic
hemorrhage	epistaxis
caustic	fracture
clinical death	rabies
brain death	EMT
heat stroke	dislocation
obstruction	debride
hypothermia	stridor
hyperthermia	911
sudden death	thorax

2. Show the videotape *Treating Medical Emergencies* (26 minutes; available from Films for the Humanities and Sciences, P.O. Box 2053, Princeton, NH 08543-2053) or the two-part videotape series *Trauma Nursing* (available from Lippincott Williams & Wilkins, 530 Walnut Street, Philadelphia, PA 19106). After the videotape presentation(s), open the class for questions and discussion.

3. Demonstrate one- and two-person CPR on a model. Have students return the demonstration during clinical laboratory on a model. Demonstrate the Heimlich maneuver. Have the students practice on a model.

4. Invite an emergency room or trauma nurse to visit the class and discuss his or her role in treating victims of trauma. After the presentation, open the class for questions and discussion.

CLINICAL

1. Invite a nurse who teaches first aid to visit the clinical laboratory and demonstrate various first aid procedures. Have the students practice first aid procedures (e.g., splinting) after the demonstration.

2. Invite a CPR instructor to visit the clinical laboratory and assist the students to be certified in CPR.

3. In the hospital setting, have the students review the policies and procedures for initiating a cardiac or respiratory code. Have the students check the unit's crash cart and replace any outdated materials.

4. In the hospital setting, ask the students to review the policies and procedures for using or disposing of hazardous materials.

SUGGESTED RESOURCES: VIDEOTAPES

Controlling violence in health care. (1994). [33 minutes]. (Available from Insight Media, P.O. Box 621, New York, NY 10024)

Ensuring infection control. (1997). [15 minutes]. (Available from Lippincott Williams & Wilkins, 530 Walnut Street, Philadelphia, PA 19106)

Infection control and universal precautions. (1992). [24 minutes]. (Available from Insight Media, P.O. Box 621, New York, NY 10024)

The ins and outs of protective barriers. (1995). [10 minutes]. (Available from Lippincott Williams & Wilkins, 530 Walnut Street, Philadelphia, PA 19106)

Patient transfer and positioning: Basic techniques for transferring patients safely. (1987). [28 minutes]. (Available from Insight Media, P.O. Box 621, New York, NY 10024)

Radiation protection. (1990). [11 minutes]. (Available from Insight Media, P.O. Box 621, New York, NY 10024)

Standards for infection control: An update for health care workers. (1995). [45 minutes]. (Available from Insight Media, P.O. Box 621, New York, NY 10024)

Surgical asepsis and sterile technique. (1993). [25 minutes]. (Available from Insight Media, P.O. Box 621, New York, NY 10024)

CHAPTER 44

Therapeutic Communication Skills

LEARNING OBJECTIVES

1. Define communication.

2. List the five components of effective communication.

3. Discuss the three parts of the communication process.

4. Explain rapport and its importance in nursing.

5. Differentiate between verbal and nonverbal communication.

6. List at least five nonverbal cues and discuss each one.

7. Discuss factors that influence the effectiveness of communication.

8. Demonstrate the interviewing and communication skills of questioning, therapeutic silence, and clarifying.

9. Modify communication skills as appropriate for the following clients: young children, older adults, nonsighted persons, hearing-impaired persons, unconscious clients, and aphasic individuals.

10. Discuss means of communicating with a client who does not speak English.

NEW TERMINOLOGY

alias	nonverbal communication
aphasia	open-ended question
body language	personal space
closed-ended question	rapport
communication	therapeutic communication
eye contact	verbal communication
interview	

KEY POINTS

- Effective communication is the cornerstone to competent nursing care. This is true in any setting.
- Communication involves a sender, receiver, channel, message, and feedback.
- Developing rapport with the client is a basic ingredient for establishing the nurse–client relationship.
- All communication has verbal and nonverbal components. Nonverbal communication is very powerful.
- Consider all personal and cultural factors about each client when communicating.
- Nurses conduct interviews to learn information about clients.
- Nurses use techniques other than words to communicate with clients who have special communication difficulties.
- Competent nursing care requires caring, accurate, and ethical communication with clients and the healthcare team.
- A nurse has the challenge to always make a positive impression when answering the telephone.
- It is important to maintain each client's confidentiality when communicating.
- Continuity of care is enhanced when thorough and accurate reporting occurs between nursing shifts.

■ Teaching–Learning Strategies

CLASSROOM

1. Using an overhead transparency as a visual aid, lead a brief discussion about the major features of the therapeutic communication process.

2. Before class, place verbal and nonverbal messages on 3 × 5 cards; assign students to portray the messages in class. Lead the class to assess the messages in light of therapeutic communication strategies.

3. Lead a brief discussion about the barriers to effective communication. Allow students to verbalize their own reactions to miscommunication.

4. Show one or more of the following videotapes: *Communicating with Clients and Colleagues: Effectiveness* (1995; available from Mosby, 11830 Westline Industrial Drive, St. Louis, MO 63146); *Effective Communication* (1995; 25 minutes; #909; available from Insight Media, P.O. Box 621, New York, NY 10024); or *Communicating with Difficult Clients and Colleagues* (1995; also available from Mosby.).

5. Provide the following CD-ROM for private use: *Communication Skills: Building Rapport and Trust* (1996; #1259; available from Insight Media, P.O. Box 621, New York, NY 10024).

CLINICAL

1. Take students to acute care, outpatient, and long-term care clinical settings and instruct them to observe types of communication as they occur.

2. Assign a client to each student and have the student complete a nursing interview using therapeutic skills at their level of understanding. Have students record their findings.

3. Allow students to evaluate their own communicating style and share results with others in postclinical conference.

4. Assist students to communicate client information to staff on their unit during the course of a clinical day.

CHAPTER 45

Admission, Transfer, and Discharge

LEARNING OBJECTIVES

1. Explain how to orient a new client to the healthcare facility.

2. Describe how to care for the client's clothing and valuable items on admission.

3. Discuss dehumanization and ways to avoid it.

4. List admission information that the nursing student or practical nurse (LPN) should report to the registered nurse (RN).

5. Demonstrate the ability to transfer the client safely and effectively.

6. Explain teaching that should occur at the time of a client's discharge from the healthcare facility.

7. Describe the procedure for discharging a client.

8. State the responsibility of the healthcare facility, the physician, and the nurse for the client who signs out of the facility against medical advice.

NEW TERMINOLOGY

dehumanization
litter scale
vital signs

KEY POINTS

- How clients feel about admission helps to determine the success of their stay in the healthcare facility.
- Clients often are apprehensive about their physical condition and about the unfamiliar procedures in the healthcare facility.
- Nurses are responsible for the initial nursing assessment.
- Clients and their belongings must be properly identified.

- Careful documentation of the admission is important to establish a baseline and to give information to other members of the healthcare team.
- When a client is transferred, explain the procedure to the client; take belongings, records, and medications; and safely transport the client.
- Discharge teaching is individual and must be documented. Make sure the client has all belongings at discharge and escort the client to the door.
- Some clients sign out of the healthcare facility against medical advice.

■ Teaching–Learning Strategies

CLASSROOM

1. Prepare an overhead transparency displaying an outline of the steps in the admission process in a healthcare facility beginning with the admitting department.

2. Lead a discussion presenting the process of admitting the client to the nursing unit; emphasize ways to prevent dehumanization during this process.

3. Allow students to share their personal experiences of being admitted to any type of healthcare facility.

4. Using an overhead transparency, present the guidelines for performing the nursing admission interview while emphasizing the practical nurse's role in this process.

5. Divide the class into two groups and assign one group to prepare to discharge Mr. S (scenario) and the other group to prepare to transfer Ms. C (scenario) to a second unit.

6. Invite a nurse to visit the class to discuss her or his experience in handling a patient who signed out of the hospital against medical advice (AMA). Distribute the AMA form obtained from a healthcare facility.

CLINICAL

1. Assign students to observe the activity in the admission department of a healthcare facility and accompany a client through the admission process.

2. Instruct the student to allow the client to express his or her feelings while being admitted to the healthcare facility.

3. Allow students to report their observations in postclinical conference.

4. Allow students to share any procedure or experience they think could have been handled differently.

5. Assign students to participate in the admission, transfer, and discharge process on the unit and document, with the guidance of faculty, on the client record.

CHAPTER 46

Vital Signs

LEARNING OBJECTIVES

1. Identify the measurements that comprise vital signs.

2. Explain reasons for changes in body temperature.

3. State normal body temperature as measured in four different body areas.

4. Define fever and its various courses.

5. Demonstrate the ability to measure temperature by the various methods discussed in this chapter.

6. Demonstrate the ability to measure and to describe radial, apical, and apical–radial pulses.

7. Demonstrate the ability to count and to describe respirations.

8. Demonstrate the ability to measure blood pressure by the various methods discussed in this chapter.

NEW TERMINOLOGY

apical pulse	orthopnea
apnea	palpation
auscultation	pedal pulse
axillary	popliteal pulse
bradycardia	pulse
Cheyne-Stokes respirations	radial pulse
crisis	rectal
cyanosis	sphygmomanometer
diastolic	stethoscope
dyspnea	systolic
fever	tachycardia
Korotkoff's sounds	tympanic
lysis	vital signs
oral	

KEY POINTS

- Temperature, pulse, respiration, and blood pressure are called vital signs (or cardinal symptoms) because they are indicators of functions of the body necessary to maintain life.
- Documentation of vital signs is essential for determining the client's status and well-being.
- Temperature is the measurement of heat inside the body. It is the balance between heat the body produces and loses.
- Pulse is the vibration of the blood through the arteries as the heart beats. It is measured by rate and rhythm.
- Respiration is the process by which the lungs bring oxygen into the body and remove carbon dioxide.
- Blood pressure measures the pressure the blood exerts on the walls of the arteries. Rate and force of heartbeat, blood vessel, condition, and blood volume determine the reading as the ventricles contract and rest.

■ Teaching–Learning Strategies

CLASSROOM

1. Prepare an overhead transparency before class with definitions of vital/cardinal signs to be displayed when the students enter the room.

2. Display a chart or overhead transparency with the normal vital signs affixed.

3. Lead a discussion about the nurse's responsibility in monitoring and documenting vital signs.

4. Have examples of the graphic record used to record the vital signs on display for students to observe.

5. Display standard equipment used to monitor vital signs available for demonstration and allow students to practice monitoring vital signs and record.

6. Show the videotape *Vital Signs* (1993; 30 minutes; available from Mosby, 11830 Westline Industrial Drive, St. Louis, MO 63146).

7. Provide time for students to demonstrate correct procedure to monitor vital signs for faculty.

CLINICAL

1. Allow students to review the policy and procedure manual for monitoring vital signs in a chosen institution (clinic, inpatient facility).

2. Take students to a busy outpatient clinic and allow them to monitor clients' vital signs as they are admitted to the clinic.

3. Have the students compare their vital sign findings with population norms.

4. At the students' level of understanding, allow them to share during postconference the ways that vital signs reflect the health status of the individual client.

CHAPTER 47

Data Collection in Client Care

LEARNING OBJECTIVES

1. Explain the role of the practical/vocational nurse in assessment and physical examination.

2. Identify common risk factors for disease and illness.

3. Define and differentiate between acute and chronic illnesses and primary and secondary illnesses.

4. Discuss the effects of inflammation and infection on the body.

5. State the rationale for obtaining a urinalysis (UA), complete blood count (CBC), urine toxicity test (UTox), and urine pregnancy test (UPT).

6. List four types of tests and procedures that primary healthcare providers use to establish a medical diagnosis. Describe how each is used in this process.

7. Discuss the purpose of the physical examination done by the primary healthcare provider and the data collected by the registered nurse or practical/vocational nurse.

8. Describe the common examination techniques of observation, inspection, palpation, percussion, and auscultation. In the skills lab, demonstrate each technique.

9. Describe common organizational formats used to perform the physical examination.

10. In the skills lab, perform a daily client data collection on a sample sheet, distinguishing between normal and abnormal findings.

NEW TERMINOLOGY

abscess
accommodation
acuity
acute disease
anergic
anorexia
auscultation
cognitive function
complication
conjunctivitis
crackle
diplopia
dysphasia
ecchymosis
emaciation
endoscope
erythema
exudate
fatigue
fissure
fistula
granulation tissue
guaiac
hemoccult
hemorrhoid
herniation
Homans' sign
hyperopia
hypoxemia
induration
infection
inflammation
inspection
kyphosis
lipoma
lordosis
macule

malaise
myopia
necrosis
nodule
observation
pallor
palpation
papule
percussion
primary disease
purulent
pustule
pyrexia
rale
rhonchi
risk factor
scoliosis
secondary disease
sequela
serosanguineous
serous
sign
smegma
strabismus
striae
stridor
suppuration
symptom
thrombophlebitis
tumor
turgor
ulcer
vesicle
wheal
wheeze
wound sinus

KEY POINTS

- Healthcare providers perform assessment and physical examination of clients for specific purposes. The primary purposes of nursing assessments are to identify and report abnormal or unusual findings, identify potential problems, and provide needed care measures within the individual nurse's scope of practice.
- Disease is a change in body structure, a definite pathological process. Illness is marked by a pronounced deviation from health, sickness, or the individual's response to change in function.
- People who are more likely to develop some diseases may have lifestyle risk factors present, such as obesity, smoking, or lack of exercise.
- People also may have a genetic or hereditary predisposition to certain physical disorders or illnesses.
- Diseases are categorized in many ways according to etiology or the effect on the person, such as acute versus chronic illness.
- Inflammation and infection are disease categories that can affect nearly every body system or part.
- Several laboratory and diagnostic tests can help primary healthcare providers to establish medical diagnoses. Nurses need a basic understanding of such procedures to provide appropriate assistance.
- The healthcare provider performs the physical examination with varying degrees of complexity and thoroughness, according to the purpose of the examination.
- The most common formats for the physical examination are the head-to-toe examination and the examination done by body systems.

■ Teaching–Learning Strategies

CLASSROOM

1. Prepare an overhead transparency or chart comparing the role of the medical doctor, the professional nurse, the practical nurse, and other professionals in performing physical examinations.

2. Lead a discussion of the risk factors of, causes of, and body's response to disease.

3. Divide the students into groups and allow them to develop a workable definition of a sign and symptom and give several examples of each. Allow them to present their findings to the class.

4. Lead a discussion to present two formats for performing a physical examination and the five techniques of examination.

5. Display some common examination tools.

6. Allow students to practice performing a head-to-toe assessment on each other while they evaluate each other's technique.

CLINICAL

1. Provide the opportunity for students to observe physical assessments being performed in the clinical setting. Allow students to share their experiences in the postconference setting.

2. Assign students to perform physical assessments for their assigned client in the healthcare setting, making appropriate documentation with faculty guidance.

CHAPTER 48

Body Mechanics and Positioning

LEARNING OBJECTIVES

1. State the three principles underlying proper body mechanics.

2. Describe safe and practical ways of assisting clients out of bed.

3. Demonstrate moving a partially or totally immobile client up in bed.

4. Explain how to move the immobile client to the side of the bed.

5. Describe and demonstrate how to transfer an immobile client from bed to chair and back.

6. Demonstrate the ability to use the wheeled stretcher (litter, gurney) safely.

7. State the purpose of range-of-motion exercises.

8. Demonstrate the ability to perform and supervise range-of-motion exercises.

9. Demonstrate the ability to position a client safely for various examinations and/or treatments.

NEW TERMINOLOGY

abduction	hemiplegia
active range of motion	inversion
adduction	isometric
base of support	line of gravity
body mechanics	logroll turn
center of gravity	paralysis
circumduction	paraplegic
(client) safety device	passive range of motion
continuous passive motion	pronation
contracture	prone
contralateral	protraction
dangling	range of motion
dorsal lithotomy (position)	recumbent (position)
eversion	retraction
extension	rotation
flexion	Sims' position
Fowler's (position)	supination
gait	transfer belt
gravital plane	transfer board
gurney	

KEY POINTS

- Pulling, pushing, or rolling an object is easier than lifting it. It requires less energy or force to keep an object moving than to start and stop it.
- Rocking backward or forward on your feet uses your body weight as a force for pulling or pushing.
- A client may become dizzy or faint when you first help him or her out of bed.
- Do not let the client grab you around the neck during transfers. Such a force can seriously injure you.
- A hospital bed should be in low position except when giving care.
- The client's body alignment when lying down should be approximately the same as if the person were standing.
- Do not force joint movement when doing PROM.
- The nurse can learn to effectively transfer and position clients for maximum safety and comfort for both nurse and client.
- The person in a safety device requires one-to-one nursing observation for safety.

■ Teaching–Learning Strategies

CLASSROOM

1. Display on an overhead transparency the underlying components of proper body mechanics.

2. Have each student drop a book on the floor and demonstrate picking the book off the floor. Indicate those who used proper body mechanics and those who did not. Allow the class to perform this same demonstration at the end of the class.

3. Lead a discussion about the use of proper body mechanics in positioning and transferring clients.

4. Demonstrate the use of mobility devices and restraints and allow the students to practice using them.

5. Show the videotape *Body Mechanics, Exercise and Activity* (1993; ISBN 0 8016 7108l; available from by Mosby, 11830 Westline Industrial Drive, St. Louis, MO 63146).

6. Allow students to practice and demonstrate positioning and transferring techniques with each other.

CLINICAL

1. Assign students to accompany and assist transport personnel in a healthcare facility and assist in transferring and transporting clients to procedures.

2. Allow students to share their experiences with the class in postclinical conferences.

3. Assign students to a comatose client in need of repositioning every 2 hours, allowing them to assist staff in repositioning the client.

CHAPTER 49

Beds and Bedmaking

LEARNING OBJECTIVES

1. State the purposes of bedmaking in the healthcare facility.

2. Demonstrate the ability to make an unoccupied, occupied, and postoperative bed.

3. Demonstrate the ability to open a bed for a client.

4. Describe the use of a bed cradle.

5. Explain the purpose of side rails.

6. Demonstrate the ability to safely adjust side rails.

7. Describe three devices that may be added to the hospital bed and their uses.

8. Identify the purposes of specialized hospital beds.

NEW TERMINOLOGY

bed cradle	occupied bed
closed bed	open bed
egg crate mattress	postoperative bed
floatation mattress	side rails
footboard	traction
mitered (corners)	trapeze

KEY POINTS

- Organize work. Gather all supplies before making the bed. Strip and make one side of the bed at a time to conserve time and energy.
- To prevent the spread of microorganisms, never shake linen or put it on the floor.
- Hold soiled linen away from your uniform, and never place soiled linen from one client's bed onto another client's bed.
- Place soiled linen in a pillow case or on a chair while continuing your work.
- A well-made bed promotes comfort and rest, helps prevent skin breakdown, and provides safety for clients.

■ Teaching–Learning Strategies

CLASSROOM

1. Have students discuss the purpose of bedmaking schedules in a healthcare facility.

2. On the chalkboard or an overhead transparency, make a list of all the equipment necessary for bedmaking.

3. Show the videotape *Bedmaking* (1993; 30 minutes; ISBN 0 8016 7096; available from Mosby, 11830 Westline Industrial Drive, St. Louis, MO 63146).

4. Provide the opportunity to practice bedmaking for occupied, unoccupied, and postoperative beds.

CLINICAL

1. Assign students to make beds on their assigned unit during clinical rotation.

2. Have students evaluate their bedmaking skills and their use of proper body mechanics.

3. Allow students to share their experiences in postclinical conference.

CHAPTER 50

Personal Hygiene and Skin Care

LEARNING OBJECTIVES

1. State at least five reasons for giving mouth care to the client.

2. In the skills lab, demonstrate assisting a client with oral care.

3. Demonstrate cleaning and caring for dentures.

4. Identify the steps involved with routine eye and ear care.

5. Demonstrate caring for the client's fingernails and toenails, addressing the reasons for attention to each area.

6. Describe how to assist clients to shave with an electric razor and with a blade razor.

7. Describe and demonstrate giving a back rub, hand/foot massage, and foot soak.

8. State three types of cleansing baths and when each one is used.

9. Demonstrate how to safely assist a client with each type of cleansing bath.

NEW TERMINOLOGY

cerumen	perineal care
halitosis	pyorrhea
nits	sordes
pediculosis	

KEY POINTS

- Oral hygiene promotes comfort, cleanliness, and nutrition.
- Personal hygiene is important to the client's self-esteem. Encourage the client to provide as much personal hygiene and self-care as possible.
- Certain conditions, such as hemorrhage, heart attack, and thrombophlebitis contraindicate vigorous rubbing of the skin and scalp.
- Shampooing the client's hair allows you to inspect the scalp for disease or injury.

- The skin is one of the body's defenses against disease and infection.
- The back rub relaxes the client and provides an opportunity for you to observe the client's skin.
- Clients need some level of skin cleansing daily. The bed bath provides an opportunity for you to observe the client's skin.

■ Teaching–Learning Strategies

CLASSROOM

1. Allow students to share their personal experiences and feelings about a time in which they were unable to perform personal hygiene for themselves.

2. Lead a discussion about the nurse's role in assisting clients in performing personal hygiene care.

3. Have a visual aid prepared (chart or overhead transparency) that outlines areas of personal care.

4. Display some of the supplies needed for performing care.

CLINICAL

1. Assign students in pairs to complete a bed bath for a totally dependent client.

2. Instruct students to perform a complete skin assessment as bathing care is provided.

3. Allow students, with faculty guidance, to document their assessment on the proper forms.

CHAPTER 51

Elimination

LEARNING OBJECTIVES

1. Describe the normal color, clarity, and odor of urine.

2. Describe at least eight abnormal patterns of urination.

3. Identify the normal color and consistency of feces.

4. Explain two deviations from normal as they relate to feces.

5. Demonstrate the techniques for assisting the client to the bathroom, giving and removing a bedpan or urinal, and transferring the client from bed to commode.

6. Explain the purpose and procedures for competent catheter care.

7. Describe techniques for relieving urinary retention.

8. List the purposes of cleansing, retention, and carminative enemas.

9. Demonstrate the technique for administering a self-contained disposable enema.

10. Describe the procedure for manual disimpaction, including a situation in which this procedure would be used.

11. Discuss nursing care for the client who is vomiting.

NEW TERMINOLOGY

anuria	fecal impaction
calculi	flatus
constipation	incontinence
Credé's maneuver	Kegel exercises
cystitis	melena
defecation	micturition
diarrhea	nocturia
dysuria	oliguria
enema	polyuria
enuresis	projectile vomiting

renal colic	urinary retention
urgency	voiding
urinary catheter	vomitus
urinary frequency	

KEY POINTS

- Adequate elimination is a basic function critical to health and life.
- Thorough handwashing and wearing of gloves are important measures when coming into contact with any body secretions or drainage from the client.
- Placing the client in as comfortable a position as possible for elimination or when vomiting and allowing for privacy are key.
- In caring for a retention catheter, precautions must be taken to prevent any source of infection from reaching the bladder.
- Diarrhea may be a symptom of impacted stool or a sign of another gastrointestinal disorder.
- Bowel and bladder continence or management can make the difference between independent living and the need for long-term care.
- Enemas may be used to assist in bowel elimination, to cleanse the bowel, or to instill medications.
- It is important to assist the client who is vomiting, to alleviate discomfort and to prevent complications.

■ Teaching–Learning Strategies

CLASSROOM

1. On a prepared overhead transparency, present the guidelines for the assessment of the function, characteristics, and pattern of elimination.

2. Describe methods of assisting with urinary and bowel elimination.

3. Show the videotapes *Catheterization and Urinary Care* (1993; ISBN 0816 7098; available from Mosby, 11830 Westline Industrial Drive, St. Louis, MO 63146).

4. Demonstrate placing a student (fully clothed) on the bedpan and allow students to practice placing one another on the bedpan using the regular and fracture bedpans.

5. Allow students to practice the skill of catheterization using anatomically correct mannequins.

6. Develop a checklist of required competencies for proper sterile technique during the catheterization procedure.

CLINICAL

1. Allow students to read the unit policy and procedure manual regarding elimination procedures.

2. Assign students to an acute care medical unit. Instruct students to become familiar with the intake and output to understand how to monitor their client's intake and output.

3. Assign students to take care of clients having elimination deficits.

4. Allow students to assess and document client elimination patterns and compare these with their normal patterns.

5. With faculty guidance, allow students to place bedpans and instill catheters and document the care given.

CHAPTER 52

Specimen Collection

LEARNING OBJECTIVES

1. Explain the purpose of monitoring a client's fluid intake and output (I&O).

2. Describe how to keep accurate I&O records.

3. Demonstrate correct measurement of urine volume and urine specific gravity, listing one medical condition associated with high specific gravity and one that is associated with low specific gravity.

4. Identify at least three reasons for laboratory examination of urine.

5. Describe and demonstrate correct collection of the following urine specimens: midstream, 24-hour, fractional, and indwelling urinary catheter.

6. Identify and explain at least one reason for collecting each of the following specimens: stool, sputum, and blood.

7. Demonstrate correct collection of a stool specimen.

8. Demonstrate correct collection of a sputum specimen.

NEW TERMINOLOGY

expectorate	occult
guaiac	specific gravity
Hemoccult	urinalysis
Hematest	urinometer
hydrometer	venipuncture

KEY POINTS

- Standard Precautions are used when collecting specimens involving any body fluids.
- Careful handwashing limits the transfer of microorganisms from one person to another and retards the spread of disease.
- Fluid intake includes all fluids consumed through the GI system (by mouth or through a tube feeding) and those fluids taken as part of IV therapy or total parenteral nutrition.

- Output includes urine and all other fluids leaving the body through any means. This includes wound drainage, emesis (vomiting), watery diarrhea, bleeding, and NG suction tube returns.
- Routine specimen collection usually is scheduled for early in the morning.
- Any specimen collected should be transported to the laboratory immediately to ensure the most accurate results.
- Urine specimens collected include single-voided, clean-catch (or midstream), catheterized, 24-hour, and fractional urine specimens.
- Stool specimens typically are evaluated for occult blood and ova and parasites.
- Sputum specimen collection requires the client to expectorate or cough up secretions from lower in the respiratory tract. The early morning specimen is the most accurate.
- Nurses do not draw blood unless they have specific education and supervised practice.

■ Teaching–Learning Strategies

CLASSROOM

1. On an overhead projector, display the following question so that students see it as they enter the classroom: "What is the nurse's responsibility related to intake and output?"

2. Obtain intake and output forms from various facilities for students to review.

3. Lead a discussion about the purpose and accurate method of measuring intake and output.

4. Display and demonstrate the use of various supplies needed to measure urine and to collect urine and stool specimens.

5. Allow students to have hands-on experience with the supplies and to verbally demonstrate their ability to use the supplies correctly.

CLINICAL

1. Assign students to care for clients on a medical unit and monitor, measure, and record intake and output accurately with faculty guidance.

2. Instruct students to review the policy and procedure manual for the collection of urine from an indwelling catheter and then allow them to perform the procedure where needed.

3. Where available, allow students to collect a variety of bodily specimens using proper technique and precautionary/safety measures. Allow students to verbalize the procedure before they perform it.

CHAPTER 53

Bandages and Binders

LEARNING OBJECTIVES

1. State at least three purposes for applying binders and bandages.

2. State the most common reasons for applying the elastic roller bandage.

3. Explain how to assess the client's extremity when it is wrapped in a bandage or has an antiembolism stocking applied.

4. Identify the most common use of the T-binder, addressing the differences when used for a male and a female client.

5. State the rationale for using Montgomery straps.

6. In the skills laboratory, demonstrate the ability to perform the following: applying all cotton elastic (ACE) bandages and antiembolism stockings and changing a dressing using Montgomery straps.

NEW TERMINOLOGY

antiembolism stockings
Kerlix
maceration
Montgomery straps
T-binder

KEY POINTS

- Elastic roller bandages may be used to encourage and support circulation after surgery. They often are used to support joints.
- Because elastic roller bandages apply direct pressure, they may be used to help control bleeding.
- When used, binders and bandages should be rewrapped every few hours. The client's skin should be assessed with each rewrapping.

- Antiembolism stockings should never be allowed to bunch or roll, which could lead to constricting circulation in the leg.
- When applying antiembolism stockings or an elastic roller bandage to an extremity, even pressure is applied over the extremity.
- The client's CMS is checked frequently when bandages are used.
- Binders are used to supply support for specific body parts. Types of binders include T-binders and abdominal binders.
- When a client requires frequent dressing changes, Montgomery straps can be used to avoid repeated tape removal and subsequent skin irritation with each dressing change.

■ Teaching–Learning Strategies

CLASSROOM

1. Display various types of bandages and binders on a table in the classroom.

2. On an overhead transparency, list the types/purposes/uses for bandages and binders.

3. Lead a discussion about the common uses for each.

4. Allow students to share personal experiences of using or wearing bandages and binders.

5. Demonstrate procedures for application of selected bandages.

6. Allow students to practice, with faculty guidance, applying bandages on each other.

7. Lead students to develop a list of assessment data for use with clients who have bandages or binders.

CLINICAL

1. Assign students to observe bandages being applied at a sports medicine clinic. Allow students to report their experiences to the group in postclinical conferences.

2. Instruct students to interview clients who have been newly bandaged and bandaged for several weeks in regard to their perception of their experience. Allow students to report findings to the group.

3. Have students assigned to care for clients with postoperative binders or bandages. Allow the students to remove and replace antiembolism stockings during routine care.

4. Guide students to perform proper assessments and documentation with faculty guidance.

CHAPTER 54

Heat and Cold Applications

LEARNING OBJECTIVES

1. State the purposes of applying heat and cold to the body.

2. Explain precautions to take when applying heat and cold.

3. Demonstrate the administration of a leg soak, sitz bath, and aquathermia pad.

4. Demonstrate the use of the cooling blanket and the application of an ice collar.

NEW TERMINOLOGY

aquathermia pad
hypothermia blanket
icecap
sitz bath
tepid sponge bath

KEY POINTS

- Heat dilates surface blood vessels.
- When heat is applied, take measures to protect the client from possible burn injury.
- Warm, moist applications heat the skin more quickly than do dry heat applications.
- Water temperature for a soak should be no higher than 105° F (41° C).
- A sitz bath applies heat and water to the pelvic or perineal and perianal area.
- Cold constricts surface blood vessels.
- Moist cold compresses are applied to small body parts.
- Tepid water sponge baths are used to reduce a client's body temperature.

■ Teaching–Learning Strategies

CLASSROOM

1. Prepare a visual aid (chalkboard or overhead transparency) displaying the types and rules for application of heat and cold therapies.

2. Display and demonstrate equipment used for these therapies, such as aquathermia pad, electric pad, heat lamp, and cold compress.

3. Lead a discussion regarding the purposes, precautions, advantages, and disadvantages of these therapies.

4. Divide students into groups and give them one specific therapy listed on a 3 × 5 card.

5. Direct them to develop a plan of care to apply this therapy (assess need for, develop a diagnostic statement, plan procedure, implement, and evaluate).

6. Allow students to choose one student in their group (see item 4) on which to apply the therapy.

CLINICAL

1. Instruct students to review the health facility's policy and procedure for heat and cold applications and report their findings in postclinical conference.

2. Assign students to clients on a medical or surgical unit to observe and apply various therapies using proper precautionary measures.

3. With faculty guidance, allow students to properly document on assessment forms.

CHAPTER 55

Client Comfort and Pain Management

LEARNING OBJECTIVES

1. Identify causes of pain.

2. Differentiate between the different types of pain.

3. Discuss the impact of chronic pain on a person's life.

4. Describe the function of endorphins in pain management.

5. Identify important considerations for assessing pain.

6. Explain the role of analgesics in pain management.

7. Name different types of analgesics and their uses.

8. Describe how surgery can provide comfort and pain relief.

9. List physical and cognitive–behavioral measures that can be used to complement pharmacologic pain management.

NEW TERMINOLOGY

acute pain	intractable pain
analgesics	neuropathic pain
chronic pain	nociception
cue	nociceptive pain
endorphins	pain threshold
guided imagery	pain tolerance

KEY POINTS

- Nociception (pain transmission) has four components: transduction, transmission, perception, and modulation.
- Acute pain (nociceptive pain) lasts for 6 months or less and is relieved once its cause is identified and treated.
- Chronic pain (neuropathic pain) lasts for more than 6 months. Common treatment measures may fail to relieve such pain.
- Factors that affect pain perception include a person's pain threshold and pain tolerance. The body's naturally occurring endorphins also influence how a person experiences pain.
- Early intervention in the cycle of pain may help control it.
- Nursing assessment of the client in pain focuses on the client's self-report of the experience and the use of pain scales.
- Pharmacology is the cornerstone of pain management.
- Surgical intervention sometimes is necessary to relieve certain kinds of pain.
- Both physical and cognitive–behavioral techniques are used to complement pharmacologic pain management.

■Teaching–Learning Strategies

CLASSROOM

1. Allow students to recall and report on their personal experiences with pain, including the cause, type, fears, concerns, and alleviating factors.

2. Have an overhead transparency prepared and display the definition of pain, causes, and types. Lead a discussion regarding this information.

3. Present an outline of the nursing assessment of pain.

4. Have students divide into six groups and develop an acronym or phrase to recall the six areas of assessing the pain experience.

5. Show the videotape *Biofeedback: Medical Application of Psycho-Physiologic Self-Regulation* (1987; 54 minutes; available from Insight Media, P.O. Box 621, New York, NY 10024).

CLINICAL

1. Take students to a healthcare facility that deals with chronic pain.

2. Allow students to observe assessments and treatments being implemented.

3. Have students interview clients who have chronic pain and participate in the nursing assessment and interdisciplinary planning of care.

4. Take students to a surgery unit in an acute care facility. Assign each student a newly postoperative client and, with faculty guidance, allow the students to complete pain assessment, management, and documentation.

5. Allow students to report their experiences in postclinical conference.

ADDITIONAL RESOURCES

Nurses Directories on: The Nurse Friendly Pain Management Nurses, website: *www.jocularity.com/directory/spec/pain.htm*
Pain Link News, website: *www.edc.org/PainLink/*

CHAPTER 56

Preoperative and Postoperative Care

LEARNING OBJECTIVES

1. Discuss classifications for determining high-risk clients.

2. List the main types of anesthetics.

3. Describe the stages of general anesthesia.

4. Explain the importance of client teaching as related to surgery.

5. List important preoperative nursing steps.

6. State the function of the recovery room and describe equipment found there.

7. Describe specific measures to take when a client returns from the post-anesthesia recovery unit.

8. Identify specific nursing actions use to alleviate postoperative pain, thirst, nausea, distension, and urinary retention and possible immediate postoperative complications.

9. Outline procedures for turning and promoting respiratory function.

NEW TERMINOLOGY

anesthesia	perioperative
atelectasis	pneumonia
dehiscence	postoperative
elective (surgery)	preoperative
emboli	splinting
evisceration	suture
hypothermia (postoperative)	thrombophlebitis
hypoxia	venous access lock
intraoperative	

KEY POINTS

- Preoperative teaching is your first line of defense against postoperative complications. Teaching also helps to make clients feel more at ease during this stressful time.

- Before giving any pre- or postoperative medication, always check the client for drug allergies.

- Early postoperative complications include hemorrhage, shock, hypoxia, and hypothermia. Be alert for early indications of these complications and respond to them quickly.

- Postoperative discomforts may include pain, thirst, abdominal distention, nausea, urinary retention, constipation, and restlessness and sleeplessness. Follow appropriate steps to alleviate the client's postoperative discomforts. Try to anticipate the client's needs based on your assessments.

- Pulmonary hygiene is extremely important in the prevention of later postoperative complications.

- Following the physician's orders for early postoperative mobility also helps to decrease the possibility of respiratory or circulatory complications.

■ Teaching–Learning Strategies

CLASSROOM

1. Divide students into four groups and lead them to develop definitions of the words *preoperative*, *perioperative*, *intraoperative*, and *postoperative*.

2. Have an overhead transparency prepared to display the types of healthcare facilities in which surgery is performed and the types of surgeries performed.

3. Lead a discussion of the assessment of a client at risk for preoperative complications.

4. Allow students to share their own experiences with surgery (negative or positive).

5. Divide students into three groups and allow them to summarize the nursing assessment and skills necessary during each phase of surgery (pre-, intra-, and postoperative).

CLINICAL

1. Take students to a same-day surgery facility to follow a client through the operative phases, making observations of the client and the staff.

2. Assign students to care for clients in a hospital the evening before surgery to participate in preoperative assessments and teaching and performing other preoperative procedures.

3. When possible, allow the student to accompany the client throughout the intraoperative and postoperative phases the next day.

4. Assign students to observe in the operating room and the postanesthesia care unit.

5. Assign students to write a paper about their observations and experiences in these areas.

ADDITIONAL RESOURCES

www.aorn.org

CHAPTER 57

Surgical Asepsis

LEARNING OBJECTIVES

1. List at least five examples of sterile and nonsterile body areas.

2. Differentiate between medical and surgical asepsis.

3. Differentiate between disinfection and sterilization.

4. List guidelines to follow when using sterile technique.

5. Demonstrate the proper technique for opening a sterile tray and a sterile package.

6. Demonstrate the correct method for handing sterile supplies to another nurse.

7. Describe the procedures for female and male catheterization.

8. Explain the procedure for removal of a retention catheter.

NEW TERMINOLOGY

autoclave	retention catheter
clean	sterile
contaminated	sterile technique
dirty	sterilization
disinfection	straight catheter
indwelling catheter	surgical asepsis

KEY POINTS

- "Clean" applies to medical asepsis. It means the removal of all gross contamination and many microorganisms.
- "Sterile" means that the item is free of all microorganisms and spores.
- When a sterile item touches anything nonsterile, it becomes contaminated.
- If a sterile item becomes contaminated or if you are unsure whether or not it is contaminated, the item is considered contaminated and must be discarded.
- Catheterization is the procedure of inserting a flexible tube through the urethra into the bladder to remove urine. This aseptic procedure requires sterile equipment and technique.
- The balloon is deflated when removing a retention catheter. The catheter is never cut for removal.
- Client and family teaching is important, especially if the client will need to perform a sterile procedure or catheter care after discharge.

■ Learning–Teaching Strategies

CLASSROOM

1. Prepare an overhead transparency displaying the definitions for asepsis: medical and surgical, disinfection, and sterilization.

2. Lead a discussion regarding the nursing skills required in the above techniques.

3. Display selected supplies and equipment used in sterile technique.

4. Demonstrate opening sterile packages and donning sterile gloves. Allow students to practice.

5. Lead a discussion about the use of catheterization during the operative phase and display equipment to be used for catheterization.

6. Show the videotape *Surgical Asepsis and Sterile Technique* (1993; 25 minutes; available from Insight Media, P.O. Box 621, New York, NY 10024).

7. Provide time for students to practice catheterization on an anatomically correct mannequin.

CLINICAL

1. Assign students to the operating room under staff supervision to observe staff performing surgical asepsis, including performing the surgical hand scrub and donning a sterile gown, gloves, mask, and boots.

CHAPTER 58

Wound Care

LEARNING OBJECTIVES

1. Identify and describe various types of wounds.

2. Describe the process of wound healing.

3. Explain the purpose of wound dressings.

4. Demonstrate changing a sterile dressing, applying a wet-to-dry dressing, and irrigating a wound.

5. Explain the causes of skin breakdown, including the causes and usual locations of pressure ulcers.

6. Describe nursing measures that help prevent skin breakdown.

7. Demonstrate assessing, cleaning, and applying medication to a pressure ulcer or other open wound.

NEW TERMINOLOGY

abrasion	laceration
debridement	pressure ulcer
decubitus ulcer	puncture
eschar	sloughing
exudate	wet-to-dry dressing
incision (surgical)	wound
ischemia	

KEY POINTS

- The skin is a barrier that protects the body's internal environment from invasion by external pathogens.
- A wound is a disruption in the skin's integrity.
- Wounds heal by first, second, or third intention.
- A dressing is applied to a wound to protect it from contamination and to collect any exudates.
- Careful sterile technique is required when dressing an open wound.
- A common cause of skin breakdown is pressure against tissues that causes ischemia and tissue death.
- Pressure ulcer prevention focuses on eliminating the causes.

- Standard Precautions are used when changing any dressing, to prevent the spread of infection to yourself or others and to avoid contaminating the wound. Wear gloves and properly dispose of all used dressings.

■ Teaching–Learning Strategies

CLASSROOM

1. Prepare an overhead transparency to present the definition of wounds and types and stages of healing.

2. Lead a discussion about the types of wound dressing.

3. Display wound dressing supplies.

4. Divide students into groups and guide them to develop a plan for performing a sterile wet-to-dry dressing change and wound irrigation. Allow each student to practice the procedure with faculty guidance.

5. Have a transparency prepared to display (with color illustrations) the four stages of pressure ulcers.

6. Divide students into four groups to discuss a means to remember the four stages of pressure ulcers.

7. Have one student sit in a wheelchair and one lie on a bed. Allow students to indicate the areas of potential skin breakdown while in these positions and develop strategies to prevent breakdown.

8. Show the videotape *Wound Care and Applying Dressings* (1993; ISBN 08016 7101; available from Mosby, 11830 Westline Industrial Drive, St. Louis, MO 63146).

CLINICAL

1. Assign students on the unit to clients requiring dressing changes and allow them to perform the procedure with faculty guidance.

2. Take students to a long-term care facility where many clients are on bed rest; have them provide care to prevent skin breakdown.

3. Assign students to clients requiring assistance in mobility and positioning.

4. Instruct students to perform skin assessments and proper positioning to prevent skin breakdown.

CHAPTER 59

Care of the Dying Person

LEARNING OBJECTIVES

1. Explain the different types of advance directives.

2. Discuss the types of codes that healthcare personnel must understand.

3. Describe the physical and emotional needs of the dying person.

4. Explain the nursing care required for the dying person.

5. Identify nursing activities that will assist the family to cope with the death of their loved one.

6. Describe the care of the body after death.

7. Discuss how members of the healthcare team can help each other cope with the death of clients.

NEW TERMINOLOGY

apnea	hyperpnea
autopsy	Kussmaul's breathing
brain death	postmortem examination
Cheyne-Stokes respiration	

KEY POINTS

- Advance directives, codes, and organ/tissue donation are three types of client wishes that nurses must be familiar with when caring for dying individuals.
- Changing the dying client's position frequently may promote comfort.
- Positioning the dying person on the side or in a semi-upright position may aid his or her breathing.
- The dying client who is incontinent needs to be kept as clean and dry as possible.
- Tube feeding or total parenteral nutrition may be instituted if the dying client is unable to eat or drink. The client may choose not to receive nourishment.
- Pain relief may be necessary to ease the dying process.
- Brain death occurs when no brain function can be identified on an EEG or by other means.
- The client's family needs nursing comfort in the form of understanding and support.
- After death, nurses give physical care to the client's body and emotional support to the family.

■ Teaching–Learning Strategies

CLASSROOM

1. Allow students to examine and share their own thoughts and experiences about death.

2. Lead a discussion about advanced directives. Display a chart or overhead transparency outlining the types of advanced directives.

3. Allow students to explore their thoughts about organ or tissue donation.

4. Display or distribute advanced directive forms and organ or tissue donation forms.

5. Lead a discussion regarding the nursing interventions necessary in caring for a dying person and the family.

6. Invite a hospice nurse to visit the class and share experiences in dealing with death and dying.

7. Review the physical signs of approaching death. Allow students to share concerns regarding assisting a client as death nears.

8. Show the videotape *Dealing with Death and Dying* (1991; 45 minutes; #314; available from Insight Media, P.O. Box 621, New York, NY 10024).

CLINICAL

1. Assign students to accompany the hospital chaplain while visiting or ministering to clients near death. Direct students to observe the chaplains while interacting with clients, their families, and the staff.

2. Instruct students to also observe the nursing staff as they interact with the client and family.

3. Assign students to visit an inpatient hospice facility and observe or assist the staff as they work with clients and their families.

4. Allow students to report their experiences to the class.

SUGGESTED RESOURCES

Ellis, J. R., Nowlis, E. A., & Bentz, P. M. (1996). *Modules for basic nursing skills.* Philadelphia: Lippincott-Raven.

Ingersoll, G. L. (1995). Licensed practical nurses in critical care areas: Intensive care unit nurses' perceptions about the role. *Heart and Lung Journal of Critical Care,* 24(1), 83–88.

Messina, J. (1997). Development and implementation of perioperative assistant training program. *AORN Journal,* 66(5), 890–904.

Priest, H., & Roberts, P. (1998). Assessing students' clinical performance. *Nursing Standard,* 12(48), 37–41.

Zimmerman, P. G. (1998). What to delegate to LPNs. *Journal of Emergency Nursing,* 24(2), 185–186.

CHAPTER 60

Review of Mathematics

LEARNING OBJECTIVES

1. Explain why an understanding of basic mathematics is essential before learning the basics of pharmacology.

2. Discuss systems of measurement used in the provision of healthcare.

3. Convert milligrams to grams and grams to kilograms.

4. Make conversions between different systems of measurement (household, metric, apothecary).

5. Demonstrate the use of ratio and proportion to calculate medication dosages.

KEY POINTS

- The metric system is the most commonly used numeric system in the world and is used for most measurements and dosages in medicine.
- The nurse must understand how to convert systems of measurement in the event a drug dosage is ordered in a different unit of measurement than is available for administration.
- Many symbols and abbreviations are used in medication orders.
- The nurse must be proficient in the use of ratios, proportions, and fractions.
- It is vital to ask if you have any questions about a medication or a dosage.

■ Teaching–Learning Strategies

CLASSROOM

1. Give students a basic math proficiency test. After scoring each student's test, determine which students need a review of basic math.

2. Show the videotape *General Medication Administration Skills* (1993; 20 minutes; available from Insight Media, P.O. Box 621,

New York, NY 10024). After the videotape presentation, review household measurements, the metric system, and the apothecary system. On 3 × 5 index cards, list various abbreviation symbols and ask students to identify their meaning during the class. These symbols should include:

mg = milligram
mcg = microgram
qt = quart
g/gm = gram
gr = grain
gtt = drop
cc = cubic centimeter
m = minim
t/tsp = teaspoon
L = liter
dr = dram
T/tbsp = tablespoon
mL = milliliter
oz = ounce
kg = kilogram
pt = pint

3. Before class, list on an overhead transparency the various household measurements from Table 60-2 in the text. Ask students to determine metric and apothecary equivalents for each household measurement.

4. Provide the students with practice problems:

   a. The physician orders Robinul 2 mg PO t.i.d. for Mr. K. You have on hand Robinul, 1-mg tablets in the container. How many will you give at one dose? In an entire 24-hour period?

   b. The physician orders for Mrs. T Hiprex 1 g PO q.i.d. after meals and at bedtime. You have on hand Hiprex 500-mg tablets. How many tablets will you give with one dose? In a 24-hour period? (More practice problems are presented in the Clinical section.)

CLINICAL

1. In the learning laboratory, show students samples of various types of medications, including medication vials, bottles, tablets, capsules, emulsions, and unit dose. Ask the students to identify the type of medication and determine its common use by referring to the *Physician's Desk Reference* or the website *www.healthsquare.com/htm.*

2. Provide the students with practice problems using fractions:

   a. $7/8 \times 3/5$ (Answer: $21/40$)
   b. $4/5 \times 1/6$ (Answer: $4/30$ or $2/15$)
   c. $3/4 \times 1/3$ (Answer: $3/12$ or $1/4$)
   d. $1/2 \times 7/9$ (Answer: $7/18$)
   e. $2/3 \times 1\frac{1}{2}$ (Answer: $2/3 \times 3/2 = 6/6$ or 1)
   f. Divide $2/3$ by $1/2$ (Answer: $4/3$ or $1\frac{1}{3}$)
   g. Divide $5/6$ by $2/3$ (Answer: $15/12$ or $1\frac{1}{4}$)
   h. Divide $1\frac{1}{2}$ by $1/3$ (Answer: $3/2 \times 3/1 = 9/2$ or $4\frac{1}{2}$)

3. Provide students with the following practice problems to calculate dosage:

   a. Physician's order reads: *Mrs. L—Lopressor, 50 mg PO b.i.d.* You have on hand Lopressor, 100-mg tablets. How much will you give in one dose?

   Answer: $1/2$ tablet

   Desired amount = 50 mg

   In what quantity = 1 tab

   Available dosage = 100 mg/per tablet

   $(50 \div 100) \times 1$ tablet = X or $1/2$ tablet in one dose

   b. Physician's order reads: *Ms. A—Penicillin G 1,200,000 units × 1 dose IM.* You have on hand Penicillin G, 600,000 units/mL. How many milliliters will you administer?

   Answer: 2 mL

   Desired amount = 1,200,000 units

   Available amount = 600,000

   In what quantity = 1 mL

   $(1,200,000 \text{ U} \div 600,000 \text{ U}) \times 1 \text{ mL} = 2 \text{ mL}$

   c. Physician's order reads: *Mr. Z—Bisacodyl 1.25 g dissolved in warm water per rectum × 1 as a cleansing enema.* The pharmacy delivers Bisacodyl 2.5 g in 1 liter of warm water. How much will you administer?

   Answer: 500 mL

   Desired amount = 1.25 g

   Available amount = 2.5 g

   In what quantity = 1,000 mL

   $(1.25 \div 2.5) \times 1,000 \text{ mL} = X$

   X = 500 mL

   d. Physician's order reads: *Mrs. B—Wellbutrin 150 mg PO b.i.d.* You have on hand 100-mg tablets. How many tablets will you administer in one dose? How much in a 24-hour period?

   Answer: $1\frac{1}{2}$ tablets per dose, 3 tablets total

   Desired amount = 150 mg

   Available amount = 100 mg

   In what quantity = 1 tablet

   $150 \text{ mg} \div 100 \text{ mg} \times 1 \text{ tablet} = X$

   24 hr dose: $1\frac{1}{2}$ tablet × 2 doses = 3 tablets

   e. Physician's order reads: *Ms. R–650 mg ASA PO t.i.d.* On hand are 325-mg/5-gr tablets. How many gr of ASA should be given in one dose?

   Answer: 10 gr or 2 tablets

   Desired amount = 650 mg

   Available amount = 325 mg or 5 gr

   In what quantity = 5 gr or 1 tablet

   $650 \text{ mg} \div 325 \text{ mg} \times 5 \text{ gr} = X$

   or $2 \times 5 = 10$ gr

   or $(650 \div 325) \times 1 = X$

   X = 2

   f. Physician's order reads: *Mr. B—Ephedrine gr 3/4.* On hand are $3/8$-gr tablets. How many tablets should be given in one dose?

   Answer: 2 tablets

   Desired amount = $3/4$ gr

   Available amount = $3/8$ gr

   In what quantity = 1 tablet

   $(3/4 \div 3/8) \times 1 = X$

   $24/12 = X$

   X = 2 tablets

   g. Physician's order reads: *Ms. G—Lomotil 1.25 mg PO PRN for diarrhea.* On hand is a liquid preparation that contains 2.5 mg/4 mL. How much should be given?

   Answer: 2 mL

   Desired amount = 1.25 mg

   Available amount = 2.5 mg

   In what quantity = 4 mL

   $1.25 \text{ mg} \times 4 \text{ mL} = 2.5 \text{ mg} \times X \text{ mL}$

   or $1.25 \div 2.5 \text{ mg} \times 4 = 2 \text{ mL}$

h. Physician's order reads: *Mr. Y—Lopid 600 mg PO b.i.d. before breakfast and dinner*. On hand are Lopid 150-mg tablets. How many tablets should be given?

Answer: 4 tablets

Desired amount = 600 mg

Available amount = 150 mg

In what quantity = 1 tablet

(600 mg ÷ 150 mg) × 1 tablet = X

i. Physician's order reads: *Mrs. C—Magnesium sulfate 5 g IM × 1 dose*. On hand is magnesium sulfate 10 g/2 mL. How many mL should be given?

Answer: 1 mL

Desired amount = 5 g

Available amount = 10 g

In what quantity = 2 mL

(5 g ÷ 10 g) × 2 mL = X

j. Physician's order reads: *Mrs. L—Nubain 10 mg IM × 1 dose*. On hand is Nubain 20 mg/1 mL. How many milliliters should be given?

Answer: 0.5 mL

Desired amount = 10 mg

Available amount = 20 mg

In what quantity = 1 mL

10 mg × 1 mL = X(20 mg)

or 0.5 mL

4. Ask the students to role-play administration of various (fake) medications and document the medication administration in a client MAR record or other chart form used for documentation of medications.

CHAPTER 61

Introduction to Pharmacology

LEARNING OBJECTIVES

1. Define the terms *medication* and *pharmacology*.

2. Explain how the Controlled Substance Act regulates specific medications.

3. Describe the proper procedure for monitoring schedule drugs in the health care facility.

4. Identify the five specific client rights related to prescribed medications.

5. List at least three drug references and one drug-related website that are commonly used by nurses.

6. Define the terms *chemical, generic, official,* and *trade names* as they refer to medications.

7. List at least five different routes of medication administration.

8. Discuss at least six factors that influence the dosage of any specific medication.

9. Differentiate between *prescribed* and *over-the-counter* medications.

10. List the seven required components of a prescription.

NEW TERMINOLOGY

agonist	official name
antagonist	paradoxical
brand name	pharmacokinetics
caplet	pharmacology
capsule	potentiating
chemical name	prescription
dosage	synergistic
enteric-coated	tablet
generic name	topical
inhalant	trade name
injectable	transdermal
medication	zydis

KEY POINTS

- Medications are substances that modify body functions. They are used to prevent disease or pregnancy, to aid in diagnosis and treatment of disease, or to restore and maintain bodily functions.
- Many laws, rules, and regulations concern the prescription, storage, and administration of medications.
- Clients have the right to know what medications they are receiving and to request available generic forms of medications. They may refuse to take medications, unless a court order exists to the contrary.
- Medication administration is a nursing task that you must take very seriously to prevent harm to clients.
- Nurses are required to know how and where to obtain information concerning medications. Several drug references and computer websites are common sources of information.
- Drugs are available in many forms, including liquids, solids, semisolids, and transdermal patches.
- Factors that affect medication dosages include the client's age, gender, weight, condition, and psychological state.
- Many medications are considered unsafe for use without a healthcare provider's supervision, and they require a specific prescription. Over-the-counter medications can be purchased by the consumer without a prescription.
- Medication orders must be carried out exactly as written. If any questions arise, the prescribing healthcare provider must be consulted for clarification. No medication can be given legally without a valid and clear order.

■ Teaching–Learning Strategies

CLASSROOM

1. Conduct a brief discussion about the federal Food, Drug, and Cosmetic Act, the United States Pharmacopeia, and the National Formulary. Ask

students to identify the purposes of the act and publications.

2. On an overhead transparency, identify the five types of controlled substances from Box 61-1 in the text. Ask students to identify each of the five drug categories. Write the students' responses on the transparency.

3. Ask students to discuss the role of the nurse in agencies with controlled substances. Ask students to role play a situation in which a nurse has forgotten to leave the narcotic keys on the unit and discovers the keys in her purse once she arrives home.

4. Ask students to identify what they should know about a particular drug before administering the drug to a client. Write the student's responses on the chalkboard or on an overhead transparency. (*Answer*: classification, use, recommended dosage, desired effects, possible adverse or untoward effects, and route of administration)

5. Ask students to compare and contrast the following related to medications: *chemical name*, *generic name*, *official name*, and *trade* or *brand name*. Ask students to list various medication forms and share their answers with the class.

6. Assign students in pairs to identify factors that influence medication dosages. Ask students to share their findings with the larger group.

7. Discuss components of a prescription medication. Ask two students to role play in class a situation in which the nurse is taking a telephone medication order from a physician. Discuss the scenario after the role-playing session.

CLINICAL

1. Before the clinical or laboratory experience, write out several prescriptions for various medications. Omit one item (e.g., client's name) from each prescription. Ask the students to identify the missing data.

2. In the clinical laboratory, have on hand various medications in several forms. Include liquids, solids, enteric coated tablets, and capsules. Ask the students to look at the various medications and identify their type.

3. In the laboratory, or computer laboratory, assign students to look up various medications using the Internet.

4. Have the students work several practice problems and role play administration of the medication to a partner. Ask the students to chart the medication after the role-playing situation.

5. Practice problems:

a. Physician's order reads: *Ms. A—Theophylline solution 160 mg PO.* You have on hand theophylline elixir 80 mg in 15 mL. How much should be given in one dose?

Answer: 30 mL

Desired amount = 160 mg

Available amount = 80 mg

In what quantity = 15 mL

160 mg ÷ 80 mg × 15 mL = X

or 2 × 15 mL = 30 mL

b. Physician's order reads: *Mr. B—Tagamet 0.8 g PO.* You have on hand Tagamet 800 mg tablets. How much will you give?

Answer: 1 tablet

Desired amount = 0.8 g

Available amount = 800 mg

In what quantity = 1 tablet

0.8 g = 800 mg

c. Physician's order reads: *Mrs. C—Tegopin solution 0.25 g.* You have on hand Tegopin 125 mg in 5 mL. How much will you give in one dose?

Answer: 10 mL

Desired amount = 0.25 g

Available amount = 125 mg

In what quantity = 5 mL

250 mg ÷ 125 mg × 5 mL = 2 × 5 mL = 10 mL

d. Physician's order reads: *Mrs. D—Depo-Provera 0.2 g.* You have on hand Depo-Provera 100 mg/1 mL. How much will you give?

Answer: 2 mL

Desired amount = 0.2 g

Available amount = 100 mg

In what quantity = 1 mL

200 mg ÷ 100 mg × 1 mL = 2 × 1 mL = 2 mL

e. Physician's order reads: *Mr. E—Diazepam 7.5 mg.* You have on hand Diazepam 5 mg in 1 mL. How much will you give in one dose?

Answer: 1¹/₂ mL

Desired amount = 7.5 mg

Available amount = 5 mg

In what quantity = 1 mL

7.5 mg ÷ 5 mg × 1 mL = 1¹/₂ × 1 mL = 1¹/₂ mL

ADDITIONAL RESOURCES

Food and Drug Administration, US Department of Health and Human Services. *www.fda.gov.*

Medication Errors, Center for Drug Evaluation and Research, Food and Drug Administration, US Department of Health and Human Services. *www.fda.gov/cder/drug/MedErrors/default.htm.*

Public Health Advisory, Center for Drug Evaluation and Research, Food and Drug Administration, US Department of Health and Human Services. *www.fda.gov/cder/drug/advisory/stjwort.htm.*

Medscape. *www.medscape.com.*

RxMED. *www.rxmed.com.*

CHAPTER 62

Classification of Medications

LEARNING OBJECTIVES

1. Describe the following classifications of medications, including the actions, possible side effects, adverse reactions, nursing considerations, and two examples of each: antibiotics, analgesics and narcotics, hypnotics and sedatives, anticonvulsants, steroids, cardiotonics, antihypertensives, and diuretics.

2. Describe client and family teaching concerning proper administration of prescribed medications.

3. Discuss the implications associated with drug-resistant bacteria.

4. Discuss the major side effects of prolonged steroid therapy.

5. Describe the most common side effects of narcotics, hypnotics, and sedatives.

6. Demonstrate the ability to accurately research information about medications.

NEW TERMINOLOGY

analgesic	diuretic
antiarrhythmic	emetic
antibiotic	expectorant
anticonvulsant	hypnotic
antihypertensive	insulin
antineoplastic	narrow spectrum
antitussive	nephrotoxicity
bactericidal	opiate
bacteriostatic	ototoxicity
broad spectrum	photosensitivity
bronchodilator	sedative
catecholamine	septicemia
cathartic	steroid
cross sensitivity	vasoconstrictor
depressant	vasodilator

KEY POINTS

- A wide variety of medications are available to treat or prevent illness or other body dysfunctions. The major groups include antibiotics, analgesics,

sedatives, anticonvulsants, and medications specific to disorders affecting each of the body systems.
- Because of the large number of medications available, the nurse must be knowledgeable in the use of drug reference books and related websites. The nurse is legally obligated to know basic information about any medication that he or she is to administer.
- Drugs are classified according to their risk to a developing fetus. However, the pregnant woman should not take any medications without medical supervision.
- In some cases, medications are prescribed even though they have undesirable side effects. Their benefits outweigh the risks and disadvantages.
- It is important to document if a client is taking any herbal supplements or using any homeopathic remedies because these can counteract or potentiate the effects of prescribed medications.
- To avoid confusion, medications often are prescribed by their generic names.

■ Teaching–Learning Strategies

CLASSROOM

1. Before class, on 3 × 5 index cards, write the following key terms:

antiarrhythmics	antihypertensive
bacteriostatic	cathartic
sedative	vasodilator
antibiotic	antitussive
bronchodilator	depressant
stimulant	bactericidal
anticonvulsant	hypnotic
catecholamine	anaphylactic
vasoconstrictor	analgesic

During the class, ask students to group themselves in pairs. Give each pair of students an index card and ask the students to define the term that appears on the card.

2. Before class, on 3 × 5 index cards, write various types of antibiotics and anti-infective agents, such as penicillins and cephalosporins. During

the class, ask students to group themselves in pairs. Distribute one or more index cards to each pair. Ask students to identify three to four medications within each category and the typical adult dosage. Ask students to share their findings with the class.

3. Before class, on an overhead transparency, list drugs classified as dermatologic agents. Ask students to provide examples for each category. Write the students' responses on the transparency.

4. Divide students into groups of three or four. Assign students a category from the drugs that affect the central nervous system. Ask students to identify two or three medications in these categories and list routes and typical adult dosages.

5. Briefly discuss epinephrine, norepinephrine, and drugs that affect the endocrine system. Assign each student one or two of these drugs to look up in the *Physicians' Desk Reference* or on an Internet site and report to the class.

6. Bring to class samples of medications for the eye and ears. During the class, distribute the sample containers and ask students to identify their use.

7. Before class, list various cardiac medications on 3 × 5 index cards. Distribute the cards in class and ask the students to identify the usual routes of administration and adult dosage, and to mention any special notes about each drug.

8. Briefly discuss medications that affect the blood, such as iron preparations and blood products. Discuss antineoplastic agents and their side effects.

9. If available, bring samples of antitussives (cough medicines), expectorants, bronchodilators, antihistamines, corticosteroids, and decongestants. Compare and contrast these medications while allowing students to view the various samples. (Most can be obtained over the counter.) Ask students to identify how many of these medications they have in their own home and share that information with the class.

10. During the class, assign pairs of students to a specific category of medications that affect the gastrointestinal system. Ask students to identify three to four medications for each category and

identify their routes and typical adult dosage. Ask students to share these findings in class and their notes about the medications. If available, bring samples (e.g., Fleet enema) to class to show the students.

11. Briefly review medications that affect the urinary and reproductive systems. Ask students to identify these medications and list the students' responses on the chalkboard or an overhead transparency.

CLINICAL

1. Before the laboratory or clinical experience, prepare small boxes or plastic bags with the names and dosages of various medications that affect specific systems. Ask students to select a box or bag and to use the *Physicians' Desk Reference* or an Internet site to look up each medication, the dosages, and use. Ask students to identify which body system their particular set of medications would affect.

2. Ask students to look at various ways of administering medications. Include various routes (e.g., intravenous, rectal) and ask students to role play administering these medications (fictitiously). After the role-playing session, ask students to document the administration of these medications in a fictitious client record or chart.

3. Give students the following practice problems:

   a. Physician's order reads: *Mr. A—Gantanol 2 g PO × 1.* You have on hand Gantanol 500-mg tablets. How much will you give in one dose? What is the purpose of this medication?

   Answer: 4 tablets. Purpose: sulfonamide/urinary tract infection

   Desired amount = 2 g

   Available amount = 500 mg

   In what quantity = 1 tablet

   2,000 mg ÷ 500 mg × 1 = 4 × 1 tablet = 4 tablets

   b. Physician's order reads: *Ms. B—Feldene 20 mg PO × 1 daily.* You have on hand Feldene 10-mg tablets. How much will you give in one dose? What is the purpose of this medication?

   Answer: 2 tablets. Purpose: anti-inflammatory/rheumatoid arthritis

   Desired amount = 20 mg

   Available amount = 10 mg

In what quantity = 1 tablet

20 mg ÷ 10 mg × 1 = 2 × 1 tablet = 2 tablets

c. Physician's order reads: *Mr. C—Serax 2 mg IM PRN.* You have on hand Serax 1 mg/1 mL. How much will you give in one dose? What is the purpose of this medication?

Answer: 2 mL. Purpose: antianxiety/used to control dangerous behavior.

Desired amount = 2 mg

Available amount = 1 mg

In what quantity = 1 mL

2 mg ÷ 1 mg × 1 mL = 2 × 1 mL = 2 mL

d. Physician's order reads: *Mrs. D—Imitrex 6 mg subQ.* You have on hand Imitrex 12 mg in 1 mL. How much will you give in one dose? What is the purpose of the medication?

Answer: 0.5 mL. Purpose: antianxiety/migraine headaches.

Desired amount = 6 mg

Available amount = 12 mg

In what quantity = 1 mL

6 mg ÷ 12 mg × 1 mL = ½ × 1 mL = ½ or 0.5 mL

e. Physician's order reads: *Miss E—Cortisone 240 mg IM × 1.* You have on hand Cortisone 120 mg/1 mL. How much will you give in one dose? What is the purpose of the medication?

Answer: 2 mL. Purpose: anti-inflammatory/arthritis.

Desired amount = 240 mg

Available amount = 120 mg

In what quantity = 1 mL

240 mg ÷ 120 mg × 1 mL = 2 × 1 mL = 2 mL

f. Physician's order reads: *Mr. F—Lente insulin 80 units subQ.* You have on hand Lente insulin 100 units/1 mL. How much will you give in one dose? What is the purpose of the medication?

Answer: 0.8 mL. Purpose: *Answer:* insulin/diabetes mellitus.

Desired amount = 80 units

Available amount = 100 units

In what quantity = 1 mL

80 units ÷ 100 units × 1 mL = 0.8 × 1 mL = 0.8 mL

g. Physician's order reads: *Ms. G—Nitrostat 0.6 mg sublingual PRN.* You have on hand Nitrostat 0.3 mg/1 tablet. How much will you give in one dose? What is the purpose of the medication?

Answer: 2 tablets. Purpose: *Answer:* antiangina/chest pain.

Desired amount = 0.6 mg

Available amount = 0.3 mg

In what quantity = 1 tablet

0.6 mg ÷ 0.3 mg = 2 × 1 tablet = 2 tablets

h. Physician's order reads: *Mr. H—Tessalon 100 mg PO t.i.d.* You have on hand Tessalon 50 mg in 5 mL. How much will you give in one dose? What is the purpose of the medication?

Answer: 10 mL. Purpose: anti-tussive/cough control.

Desired amount = 100 mg

Available amount = 50 mg

In what quantity = 5 mL

100 mL ÷ 50 mg × 5 mL = 2 × 5 mL = 10 mL

i. Physician's order reads: *Mrs. I—Zantac 150 mg b.i.d. PO and 300 mg HS daily.* You have on hand Zantac 300 mg/tablet. How much will you give in one b.i.d. dose? How many total tablets per day? What is the purpose of this medication?

Answer: ½ tablet b.i.d.; 2 tablets total. Purpose: GI drug/ulcers and gastric acid reflux.

Desired amount = 150 mg

Available amount = 300 mg

In what quantity = 1 tablet

150 mg ÷ 300 mg = ½ × 1 tablet = ½ tablet b.i.d.

Total: ½ + ½ + 1 tablet = 2 tablets

CHAPTER 63

Administration of Medications

LEARNING OBJECTIVES

1. Explain how medications are stored in healthcare facilities.

2. Discuss the importance of documenting medication administration in the medication administration record (MAR), the computerized record, or the client's chart.

3. Differentiate among STAT, PRN, and HS medications.

4. Discuss the importance of the "five rights" of medication administration, including steps to observe before administering medications.

5. Differentiate between desired and undesired effects and local and systemic medication effects.

6. Explain what is meant by enteral and parenteral administration.

7. Demonstrate various methods of enteral medication administration.

8. Demonstrate the proper technique for administering subcutaneous, intramuscular, and intradermal injections.

9. Identify nursing considerations for the use of total parenteral nutrition.

10. Discuss the use of infusion pumps, piggyback administration of medications, and intermittent infusion devices such as heparin or saline locks.

NEW TERMINOLOGY

ampule
anaphylactic effect
anergic
diluent
enteral
heplock
infiltration
infusion
medication administration
   record
ophthalmic
otic
parenteral
transfusion
vial
z-track

KEY POINTS

- Because the administration of medications is perhaps the single most important and potentially dangerous nursing function, follow the rules of safe administration precisely.
- The "five rights" of administration are the right client, right medication, right dosage, right time, and right route.
- Document all medications after you administer them.
- Local effects of a medication are restricted to the area in which they are administered. Topical medications usually have local effects. Systemic effects mean that a medication's effects spread throughout the body.
- STAT medications are to be given immediately; PRN medications are given as needed; HS medications are PRN medications that are given at bedtime to help clients sleep.
- Enteral administration means through the gastrointestinal system (most commonly this is considered to be PO or via NG tube). Parenteral administration means administration through any other method and most commonly refers to administration by some type of injection.

- Enteral medication administration methods include oral, sublingual, buccal, and through a gastric tube. Rectal administration technically is considered enteral administration.
- Proper technique and site preparation for intradermal, subcutaneous, intramuscular injections, and IV are essential.
- Monitoring of IV infusion solutions, rates, and sites must be done at least every hour. The insertion site must be kept as clean and dry as possible.

■ Teaching–Learning Strategies

CLASSROOM

1. Ask students to define the following terms:

ampule	vial
anaphylactic effect	vastus lateralis
enteral	subcutaneous
intradermal	sublingual
toxicity	suppository
ventrogluteal	infiltration
intramuscular	transfusion
intravenous	total parenteral
infusion	nutrition
medication administration record (MAR)	deltoid

Write the students' responses on an overhead transparency or the chalkboard.

2. Show one or more of the following videotapes: *Administering Injectable Medications* (1993; 14 minutes; #XU647); *Administering Injectable Medications* (1996; 20 minutes; #XU1610); or *Administering Medications by Injection* (1993; 20 minutes; #XU648; all available from Insight Media, P.O. Box 621, New York, NY 10024). After the videotape presentation(s), open the class for discussion.

3. Conduct a brief discussion with the class about the proper methods of storing medications and review the following terms: STAT, PRN, IV, OTC, and HS.

4. Ask students to identify "safety in administration of medications." Write the students' responses on the chalkboard or overhead transparency.

5. Show the videotape *The Nurse's Guide to Enteral Feeding Tubes* (1993; 32 minutes; available from Insight Media, P.O. Box 621, New York, NJ 10024). After the videotape presentation, open the class for discussion.

6. Show the videotape *Intravenous Medications* (1993; 30 minutes; available from Lippincott Williams & Wilkins, 530 Walnut Street, Philadelphia, PA 19106). After the videotape presentation, open the class for discussion.

7. Briefly review the role of the LPN in caring for clients with TPN.

CLINICAL

1. In the learning laboratory, place the students in pairs. Provide equipment for administration of subcutaneous, intramuscular, and intravenous medications. After a demonstration of each skill, allow students to practice calculating dosages, preparing the medications, and calculating intravenous flow rates.

2. Briefly review the procedure for setting up medications. Allow students to practice documentation of medications given to a fictitious client.

3. Ask two students to volunteer a role-playing situation in which a client refuses a medication and another in which the nurse has made a medication error. Ask students for feedback after the role-playing situation.

4. Provide students with practice medication problems such as the following:

   a. Physician's orders read: *Mr. A—Meperidine 50 mg IM PRN for pain.* You have on hand Meperidine 25 mg per mL. How much will you give? What is the purpose of this medication?

   Answer: 2 mL. Purpose: narcotic—alleviation of pain.

   Desired amount = 50 mg

   Available amount = 25 mg

   In what quantity = 1 mL

   50 mg ÷ 25 mg = 2 × 1 mL = 2 mL

b. Physician's order reads: *Ms. B.—Morphine sulfate 10 mg IM PRN for pain.* You have on hand Morphine sulfate 15 mg per 1 mL. How much will you give? What is the purpose of this medication?

Answer: ²⁄₃ mL or 0.66 mL. Purpose: narcotic—alleviation of pain.

Desired amount = 10 mg

Available amount = 15 mg

In what quantity = 1 mL

10 mg ÷ 15 mg = ²⁄₃ × 1 mL = ²⁄₃ mL or 0.66 mL

c. Physician's order reads: *Mr. C.—Tagamet (cimetidine) 150 mg IM STAT.* You have on hand Tagamet 300 mg per 2 mL. How much will you give? What is the purpose of this medication?

Answer: 1 mL. Purpose: decrease gastric secretions.

Desired amount = 150 mg

Available amount = 300 mg

In what quantity = 2 mL

150 mg ÷ 300 mg = ½ × 2 mL = 1 mL

SUGGESTED RESOURCES

Administering medications by nonparenteral routes. (1993). [Videotape, 20 minutes]. (Available from Insight Media, P.O. Box 621, New York, NY 10024)

Avoiding medication errors. (1989). [Videotape, 30 minutes]. (Available from Insight Media, P.O. Box 621, New York, NY 10024)

Calculate with care. (1984). [CAI]. (Available from Lippincott Williams & Wilkins, 530 Walnut Street, Philadelphia, PA 19106)

Clinical pharmacology. (1996). [CD-ROM]. (Available from Insight Media, P.O. Box 621, New York, NY 10024)

Introduction to parenteral medications. (1990). [Videotape; 23 minutes]. (Available from Lippincott Williams & Wilkins, 530 Walnut Street, Philadelphia, PA 19106)

Understanding medication guidelines. (1996). [Videotape; 15 minutes]. (Available from Insight Media, P.O. Box 621, New York, NY 10024)

CHAPTER 64

Normal Pregnancy

LEARNING OBJECTIVES

1. Define the key terms related to pregnancy and gestation.

2. Identify the components of preconceptional care and state five nursing considerations related to preconceptional care.

3. Describe the process of conception, implantation, and placental development.

4. Differentiate at least five major events of the development of the embryo and the growth of the fetus.

5. Describe the structure and functions of the placenta, umbilical cord, fetal membranes, and amniotic fluid.

6. Outline the pathway of fetal blood circulation.

7. Contrast the presumptive, probable, and positive signs of pregnancy. State at least three nursing considerations for each.

8. Describe changes in a woman's anatomy and physiology that occur during each trimester of pregnancy.

9. Discuss anticipatory guidance for pregnant women related to changes in the body's structure and function.

10. Identify at least five client teaching concepts related to prenatal care.

11. Prepare a nursing care plan that teaches healthy lifestyle behaviors for pregnant women.

12. Identify recommended nutritional guidelines during pregnancy.

13. Describe at least five common discomforts of pregnancy, how they might be alleviated, and how a woman can differentiate them from more serious problems.

14. Prepare a nursing care plan for a client who is expecting her first child. Explore ways to support the process of preparing for parenthood and an expanding family.

NEW TERMINOLOGY

amnion	implant
amniotic fluid	lactation
antepartum	linea nigra
anticipatory guidance	lordosis
ballottement	melasma
cephalocaudal	morula
Chadwick's sign	multifetal
chorion	Nägele's rule
colostrum	nurse-midwife
conception	obstetrician
congenital	obstetrics
decidua	para/parity
doppler	pica
ductus arteriosus	placenta
ductus venosus	preconception
embryo	prenatal
fetoscope	primigravida
fetus	ptyalism
fundal height	quickening
gestation	trimester
Goodell's sign	ultrasound
grand multipara	umbilicus
gravid/gravida	viable/viability
Hegar's sign	Wharton's jelly
hyperemesis gravidarum	zygote

KEY POINTS

- Gravida refers to the number of pregnancies a woman has had; para refers to the outcome of those pregnancies.
- Preconception care includes addressing woman's habits, nutrition, psychosocial needs, and risks associated with medications, diseases, and genetic defects.
- The fertilized ovum, or zygote, eventually develops into the fetus and all supporting structures: placenta, membranes, and umbilical cord.
- The period of the embryo is the critical period of human development, when the organs and systems are formed; the period of the fetus is a period of further growth and development.
- The maternal and fetal blood does not mix under normal circumstances; the placenta provides a

place for exchange of gases, nutrients, and fluid between the mother and the fetus.

- In fetal circulation, oxygenated blood travels from the placenta through the umbilical vein, whereas deoxygenated blood is carried from the fetus to the placenta through the two umbilical arteries.
- Only the positive signs of pregnancy prove there is a fetus.
- A woman's body changes in both structure and function because of the size of the growing fetus and the hormones produced during pregnancy.
- Anticipatory guidance about the changes that are coming with pregnancy gives a woman or a couple time to prepare for those changes.
- A healthy lifestyle for a pregnant woman includes maintaining adequate nutrition, avoiding harmful substances, and exercising.
- Good nutrition during pregnancy is dependent upon the mother taking in enough calories to provide energy and enough protein to support herself and the rapidly growing fetus, as well as consuming the recommended amount of vitamins and minerals every day.
- All pregnant women should gain weight; the amount that is ideal for each woman is based on her height and weight before the pregnancy.
- The common discomforts of pregnancy do not threaten the health of the mother or the fetus but may be similar to warning signs of more serious problems. It is important to know how to distinguish common discomforts from warning signs and report them as necessary.
- The physiologic changes of pregnancy are just as tremendous as the physical changes; every woman and family deserves support in dealing with these changes.

■ Teaching–Learning Strategies

CLASSROOM

1. Ask students to define the following terms:

para	trimester
amnion	gravida
gestation	conception
antepartal	embryo
ballottement	linea nigra
hydramnios	viability
quickening	midwife
hyperemesis	fetus
gravidarum	placenta
teratogen	estimated date of
chloasma	confinement

Write the students' responses on the chalkboard or an overhead transparency.

2. Show the videotape *Examination of the Pregnant Woman* (1987; 20 minutes; available from Lippincott Williams & Wilkins, 530 Walnut Street, Philadelphia, PA 19106; ISBN 0-397-56693-X). After the videotape presentation, open the class for discussion. Use the instructor's manual provided with the videotape for additional discussion.

3. Before class, make a transparency of the fetal circulation. During the class, trace fetal circulation using the transparency.

4. Use the drawings to conduct a discussion about various stages of fetal development.

5. Before class, using 3 × 5 index cards, write one minor discomfort of pregnancy (e.g., nausea and vomiting) on each card. During the class, divide students in pairs. Distribute one or more index cards to the pairs and ask them to outline nursing interventions (teaching) for each discomfort of pregnancy.

6. Ask students to differentiate presumptive, probable, and position signs of pregnancy. Write the students' responses on the chalkboard or an overhead transparency.

7. Invite a dietitian to visit the class and discuss the nutritional needs of a pregnant client. After the presentation, open the class for discussion and questions.

CLINICAL

1. Assign pairs of students to visit an antepartal clinic and observe a nurse working in the clinic. Ask students to share their experiences with the larger group.

2. Assign pairs of students to attend one or more preparation-for-parenting classes. Ask students to write a one-page report on their observations during the class.

3. Ask students in pairs to design a poster that focuses on care during pregnancy. Students can focus on drug use, nutrition, or one of the minor discomforts. Ask the students to bring their

posters to clinical conference. After the presentation, offer to donate the students' posters to an antepartal clinic.

4. Ask students to interview a pregnant client about her pregnancy. Ask students to share their interview findings with the larger group.

CHAPTER 65

Normal Labor, Delivery, and Postpartum Care

LEARNING OBJECTIVES

1. Identify at least three choices or options for locations for birth. Discuss at least two advantages and disadvantages for each option. Identify at least two nursing considerations for each choice.

2. Define and give at least four differences between true labor and false labor. State at least two nursing considerations related to each type of labor.

3. Explain the significance of lightening, Braxton-Hicks contractions, effacement, dilation, "show," spontaneous rupture of membranes (SROM), artificial rupture of membranes (AROM), engagement, nulliparous, and parous.

4. Differentiate between the following events that occur during contractions: increment, acme, decrement, rest interval, frequency, duration, intensity, and length of relaxation time.

5. Define and discuss at least three nursing considerations for each of the following terms: lie, presentation, station, and position.

6. Discuss the events that indicate the onset of the first stage of labor.

7. Differentiate between the three phases of the first stage of labor. Identify at least three nursing considerations for the latent phase, the active phase, and the transitional phase.

8. Identify the events of the second stage of labor and the significance of bearing down and crowning. Identify at least three nursing considerations related to this stage.

9. Identify the events of the third stage of labor and explain the significance of the expelled placenta. Identify at least three nursing considerations related to this stage.

10. Identify the events of the fourth stage of labor and explain the significance of involution. Identify at least three nursing considerations related to this stage.

11. Compare the advantages and disadvantages of at least four comfort measures related to contractions. State at least four nursing considerations related to epidural and general anesthesia.

12. Discuss at least four nursing considerations related to external fetal monitoring.

13. Differentiate between the following terms: *acceleration, decelerations, early decelerations, late decelerations,* and *decreased variability.*

14. Identify at least three nursing responsibilities to the newborn and the mother immediately after birth.

15. Define and differentiate between the following terms: *lochia rubra, lochia serosa,* and *lochia alba.* State at least three nursing considerations for each.

16. In the nursing skills lab, demonstrate the techniques of postpartum care, including fundal massage, episiotomy and perineal assessment, peripad changes, Homans' sign, and bladder assessment.

17. In the nursing skills lab, present a client teaching session on the advantages of breastfeeding. Include the following concepts: *colostrum, lactation, let-down reflex, engorgement,* and *expression of milk.*

18. Discuss the chances of becoming pregnant when a woman is breastfeeding. Differentiate between the return of menstruation and ovulation.

NEW TERMINOLOGY

after-pains	intrapartum
amniotomy	involution
Braxton-Hicks contractions	labor
cervical os	labor contractions
colostrum	lactation
crowning	lightening
dilation	lochia
effacement	nuchal cord
engorgement	postpartum
episiotomy	show
fetal monitor	

KEY POINTS

- The role of the labor and delivery nurse is to ensure maternal and fetal well-being.
- The onset of true labor may be difficult to recognize, even for the multigravida.
- Rhythmic uterine contractions causing cervical dilation and effacement and descent of the fetal presenting part characterize true labor.
- Normal labor has four distinct, sequential stages. In the first stage cervical dilation and effacement occur, along with fetal descent. The second stage is the birth of the newborn. The third stage is the delivery of the placenta. Family bonding, maternal recovery, and infant stabilization occur in the fourth stage.
- An important nursing responsibility during labor is assessing frequently to keep the birth attendant informed of the woman's progress and any deviations from normal for the woman or fetus.
- The fetal heart rate can be heard and assessed using a fetoscope, Doppler ultrasound device, or electronic fetal monitor.
- Various patterns of fetal response to uterine activity can be identified with electronic fetal monitors, and appropriate interventions can be started early.
- Lacerations may occur, even during the "normal" labor and delivery process.
- The fourth stage of labor is a critical time for the mother and her newborn. The major concerns during this time are preventing maternal hemorrhage and maintaining the newborn's respiratory and cardiac function.
- In the postpartum woman, major changes (involution) occur in most body systems, restoring them to their normal prepregnant state.
- The uterus decreases in size, the placental site and episiotomy heal, and lochia progresses from rubra to alba during the 6 weeks after delivery.
- Breasts will begin producing milk within 3 to 5 days after delivery.

- Lactation may be suppressed by mechanical means, such as ice packs and compression binders, and by avoiding breast stimulation. Medications usually are not used because the risks outweigh the benefits.
- Client teaching regarding fundal height and consistency, lochia, perineal care, nursing and breast changes, uterine cramping, backache, and fatigue are essential concepts for the new mother to learn.

■ Teaching–Learning Strategies

CLASSROOM

1. Ask students to define the following terms:

effacement	episiotomy
dilatation	crowning
lightening	intrapartum
after-pains	postpartum
engorgement	os
lochia	labor
station	lactation
lie	crowning
position	show
amniotomy	involution
colostrum	

Write the students' responses on the chalkboard or on an overhead transparency.

2. Show the videotape *Human Birth* (1974; 23 minutes; available from Lippincott Williams & Wilkins, 530 Walnut Street, Philadelphia, PA 19106). After the videotape presentation, open the class for discussion and questions.

3. Conduct a discussion about true versus false labor. Ask students to differentiate between true and false labor and write their responses on the chalkboard or on an overhead transparency.

4. Discuss the three phases of the first stage of labor. Ask the students to identify components of each phase and the nursing care required.

5. On an overhead transparency or the chalkboard, write "Danger Signs of Labor." Ask students to list the danger signs of labor.

6. Briefly review internal and external fetal monitoring. Ask students to identify the nursing

care required for early, variable, and late deceleration patterns.

7. Outline nursing care for the second stage of labor and immediate care of the newborn. Ask students to share their own experiences with the birth process.

8. Review immediate and later postpartum care needs and teaching aspects. Ask students to identify the signs of postpartum hemorrhage.

CLINICAL

1. Assign students to a clinical setting that has a labor, delivery, and postpartum unit. Ask students to work with the nursing staff in caring for clients in various stages of the labor, delivery, and postpartum process. Ask students to share their observations during clinical conference.

2. In the clinical laboratory, show the videotape *Childbirth and Infant Care* (available from Nimco, Inc., P.O. Box 9, 102 Highway 81 North, Calhoun, KY 42327; #NIM-SM-HAB4-V7). After the videotape presentation, open the class for discussion and questions.

3. Assign students to a nurse-midwife clinic, if available. Ask the students to spend the day with the nurse-midwife. Ask students to compare routine hospital deliveries with care by a nurse-midwife. Ask students to share their observations with the larger group.

4. If possible, assign one or two students to observe a cesarean section and work with a nurse during the recovery period. Ask students to compare the care for a client with a vaginal delivery to a client who has experienced a cesarean section. Ask students to share their findings with the larger group.

CHAPTER 66

Care of the Normal Newborn

LEARNING OBJECTIVES

1. Describe the respiratory and cardiovascular changes that occur in the newborn during the transition from the fetal to the newborn environment.

2. Identify the four causes of newborn heat loss. State at least one example of each. Identify at least two nursing considerations related to prevention of cold stress of the neonate.

3. State the four main goals for immediate care of the newborn.

4. Identify the five components of the APGAR score. Identify at least two nursing considerations related to each component.

5. Discuss the procedure for proper identification of the newborn. State at least three nursing considerations related to safety precautions, prevention of nosocomial infections, and completion of birth documentation.

6. State at least two nursing considerations related to universal precautions, eye prophylaxis, vitamin K administration, and parental bonding.

7. Discuss the normal ranges of weight and length of the neonate. State at least two nursing considerations related to molding, caput succedaneum, cephalhematoma, anterior fontanel, and posterior fontanel.

8. Define and discuss at least two nursing considerations related to the following terms: pseudomenstruation, phimosis, acrocyanosis, milia, Epstein's pearls, erythema toxicum, petechiae, Mongolian spots, lanugo, and vernix caseosa.

9. Define the following reflexes of the newborn: rooting, palmar grasp, Moro, tonic neck, Babinski, stepping, and sucking.

10. Identify at least 10 elements of information regarding the process of labor and birth that must be reported to the newborn nursery nurse.

11. Identify the components of the initial assessment of a newborn. Include at least two nursing considerations related to the umbilical cord, physical measurements, vital signs, respiratory status, elimination, and meconium.

12. Identify the components of a routine assessment of a newborn. Include at least two nursing considerations related to vital signs, weight, urine, and stools.

13. State at least three nursing considerations related to each of the following: holding a newborn, dressing a newborn, cord care, circumcision, and sleep.

14. State the nine main benefits of breastfeeding.

15. Define the following terms: colostrum, foremilk, hindmilk, and LATCH. Identify at least two nursing considerations for each term.

16. State at least two nursing considerations related to the following common problems of breastfeeding: sore and cracked nipples, engorgement, plugged ducts, and mastitis.

17. Identify at least three teaching considerations regarding nutrition for the breastfeeding mother.

18. Identify at least three teaching considerations for the mother who is bottle feeding.

NEW TERMINOLOGY

acrocyanosis	hypothyroidism
alveoli	lanugo
bonding	mastitis
brown fat	meconium
canthus, inner and outer	milia
caput succedaneum	molding
cephalhematoma	Mongolian spots
circumcision	neonate
desquamate	ophthalmia neonatorum
en face position	phimosis
epispadias	port-wine stain
Epstein's pearls	prepuce
erythema toxicum	pseudomenstruation
fontanels	smegma
foremilk	stork bites
galactosemia	surfactant
hindmilk	vernix caseosa
hypospadias	

KEY POINTS

- The Apgar score is used for immediate assessment of the newborn based on heart rate, respiratory effort, muscle tone, reflex irritability, and color. The maximum score is 10. The evaluation is done at 1 minute after birth and again at 5 minutes. An Apgar score of 7 or less indicates a need for neonatal resuscitation.
- Newborns can lose heat by convection, conduction, radiation, and evaporation.
- To prevent cold stress; the nurse should keep the neonate dry, provide a hat or cap to prevent heat loss from the head, provide a heat source for the neonate until his/her temperature stabilizes (skin-to-skin contact with a parent, isolette, or radiant warmer), and maintain the room temperature at about 75° F.
- At the time of delivery, neonatal assessments include the Apgar score, additional evaluation of the need for resuscitation, temperature regulation, and neonatal adaptation to life outside the uterus.
- When an infant is admitted to the nursery, ongoing assessments include evaluation of respiratory status, temperature regulation, umbilical cord, body measurements, and elimination.
- Daily newborn assessments include weight, respiration, elimination, and feeding. Each of these items should be reviewed at the time of discharge.

- Newborn identification is essential to ensure that the mother goes home with her own baby.
- Identification measures used in many hospitals include matching identification bands, taking footprints, using electronic bracelets, and keeping an accurate and complete hospital record. The identification should be confirmed each time the mother and neonate are brought together and again at hospital discharge.
- The normal newborn has a respiratory rate of less than 60 beats per minute, a heart rate of 110 to 150 beats per minute, and a normal body temperature. The neonate may have a variety of temporary or permanent skin markings. The effects of maternal hormones on the neonate's breasts and genitals may last for a few weeks.
- When weighing an infant, care should be taken to avoid cold stress; the infant must never be left alone. In measuring the infant, use the crib sheet to mark where the crown of the head is, then stretch the legs, make another mark, and measure between the marks.
- Daily care of the neonate includes cord care, skin care, assessment of possible problems, and attention to the neonate's need for security, safety, and bonding with the parents.
- A circumcised male neonate needs frequent changes of a sterile dressing over the wound and assessment for complications; he should not be laid on his stomach.
- Normal newborn stools progress from meconium to transitional stools as feeding begins. Breastfed neonates have loose, yellow stools; neonates drinking formula have more firm stools that may be darker.
- The breastfeeding mother needs information regarding helping the neonate latch on; taking care of the nipples; alternating breasts; using different positions; and recognizing complications.
- Bottle-fed neonates should be held during feedings. The bottle should not be propped or the neonate left unattended.
- All neonates should be bubbled during and after feeding. This can be accomplished by sitting the neonate on your lap, holding the neonate on your shoulder, or laying the neonate across your knees and gently patting his or her back until bubbling occurs. Some spit-up is normal.

■ Teaching–Learning Strategies

CLASSROOM

1. Ask the students to define the following terms:

acrocyanosis	pseudomenstruation
circumcised	caput succedaneum
phenylketonuria	lanugo
Apgar score	smegma
desquamate	cephalhematoma
phimosis	meconium
bonding	vernix caseosa
fontanels	transitional stool
pseudo	engorgement
caput	plugged ducts
galactosemia	mastitis

2. During class, show the videotape *Physical Assessment of the Normal Newborn,* 2nd edition (1992; 27 minutes; ISBN 0-397-56782-0; available from Lippincott Williams & Wilkins, 530 Walnut Street, Philadelphia, PA 19106). After the videotape presentation, open the class for discussion and questions.

3. Briefly review the Apgar scoring method. Ask students to identify symptoms of respiratory distress in a newborn and resuscitation of a newborn. Write the students' responses on the chalkboard or on an overhead transparency.

4. Briefly review immediate and daily routine care of the newborn. Ask students to share their personal experiences with the class.

5. Invite a mother who is involved with La Leche League to visit the class and discuss breastfeeding. After the presentation, open the class for questions and discussion.

CLINICAL

1. Assign students to observe in a delivery room setting during a birth. Ask students to identify immediate newborn care needs. Ask students to observe the staff performing resuscitation of a newborn.

2. Assign students to a newborn admission nursery. Demonstrate the procedure for assessing a neonate, weighing a newborn, bathing a newborn, and performing a PKU blood draw. Assign students to a newborn and ask them to perform a neonatal assessment and the other procedures. Ask students to share their observations with the larger group.

3. Before the clinical experience, ask students to develop a teaching plan related to newborn care for a first-time mother. Assign students to a first-time mother in the clinical setting and ask students to carry out their teaching plan.

4. Assign several students to clients who are bottle feeding their newborns. Ask students to assist their clients with newborn nutrition needs.

5. Assign students to a nurse in the clinical setting who is doing the discharge teaching of a postpartum family. Ask students to identify other teaching needs and the potential need for follow-up care by a home visit or clinic visit. Ask students to share their observations with the larger group.

CHAPTER 67

High-Risk Pregnancy and Childbirth

LEARNING OBJECTIVES

1. Explain the term *high-risk pregnancy*.

2. Define and differentiate between the following tests used to assess fetal status: amniocentesis, ultrasound scanning, OCT, NST, FBP, PUBS, CVS, and MSAFP.

3. Define and differentiate between the following types of abortions: threatened, complete, septic, recurrent spontaneous, inevitable, incomplete, missed, and induced or therapeutic. State at least three nursing considerations for each.

4. State at least three nursing considerations for an ectopic pregnancy.

5. Describe the events leading to gestational trophoblastic disease and state at least three nursing considerations related to the outcome of this condition.

6. Discuss at least five implications to mother and fetus when hyperemesis gravidarum exists.

7. Define PIH, mild and severe preeclampsia, and eclampsia. State at least three nursing considerations for each condition.

8. Discuss at least five nursing implications related to a pregnant woman with existing diabetes mellitus.

9. State at least three nursing implications related to the pregnant woman with an existing cardiac disorder or who has a chemical dependency.

10. Define and discuss the following disorders: maternal infection, Rh sensitization, erythroblastosis fetalis, ABO incompatibility, and polyhydramnios. State at least three nursing concerns for each condition.

11. Define and differentiate between placenta previa, abruptio placentae, and placenta accreta. State at least three nursing considerations for each condition.

12. Discuss at least three of the nursing implications related to prolonged pregnancy, multiple pregnancy, adolescent pregnancy, and pregnancy in the woman older than 40 years.

13. Develop a nursing care plan for a client with the following complications: maternal hemorrhage, premature rupture of membranes (PROM), preterm labor, precipitate labor and delivery, uterine rupture, uterine inertia and fetal dystocia, cephalopelvic disproportion (CPD), and abnormal fetal presentations.

14. Define and differentiate at least three aspects of nursing care related to a prolapsed cord and a nuchal cord.

15. Discuss at least three nursing considerations related to the induction of labor with drugs or amniotomy.

16. Discuss at least three nursing considerations related to version, forceps delivery, and vacuum extraction.

17. Discuss at least three nursing considerations related to preoperative care and postoperative care after a cesarean delivery. Identify at least three special considerations related to care of the newborn.

18. Identify and discuss the common complications of the postpartum period, including postpartum hematoma, postpartum hemorrhage, uterine atony, thrombophlebitis, puerperal infection, cystitis, and mastitis.

19. Define and differentiate between postpartum blues, depression, and psychosis.

20. In the skills lab, use therapeutic communications to role-play a scenario in which a newborn has died.

NEW TERMINOLOGY

ABO incompatibility
abruptio placentae
amniocentesis
amniotomy
atony
breech
cerclage
cesarean delivery
choriocarcinoma
cystitis
delivery forceps
dystocia
eclampsia
ectopic
erythroblastosis fetalis
gestational diabetes
high risk pregnancy
hydatidiform mole
hydramnios
hyperemesis gravidarum
induction

macrosomia
mastitis
nuchal cord
placenta accreta
placenta previa
polyhydramnios
postpartum hematoma
postpartum hemorrhage
preeclampsia
premature cervical dilation
products of conception
prolapsed cord
puerperal
station
stress test
thrombophlebitis
transverse lie
uterine inertia
vacuum extraction
version
vertex

KEY POINTS

- A high-risk pregnancy is one in which complications of the pregnancy or preexisting health conditions endanger the life or well-being of the woman or fetus.
- Some spontaneous abortions occur for unknown reasons; however, fetal maldevelopment and certain maternal factors account for many cases. The type of spontaneous abortion dictates medical and nursing management.
- Ectopic pregnancy is a significant cause of maternal morbidity and mortality.
- A healthcare facility discharges a woman with hyperemesis gravidarum when she regains fluid and electrolyte balance and begins to gain weight.
- Careful management of pregnancy-induced hypertension is crucial.
- Existing medical disorders, such as diabetes mellitus, cardiac disorders, and chemical dependency, will complicate pregnancy and require special care.
- Insulin requirements in the woman with insulin-dependent diabetes increase as the pregnancy advances. Control of maternal blood glucose is essential for preventing hydramnios, dystocia, and other complications.
- Premature separation of the placenta and placenta previa are differentiated by the type of bleeding, uterine tonicity, and the presence or absence of pain.

- Diagnostic techniques for assessing fetal status include amniocentesis, ultrasound, nonstress testing, oxytocin challenge testing, and biophysical profile.
- Complications of labor and delivery are related to the status of the membranes, the pace of labor, the effectiveness of contractions, the passageway, and the passenger.
- Dystocia is active labor that does not result in effective cervical dilation or effacement.
- Operative obstetrics concerns procedures that involve manipulating the fetus to facilitate birth. Version, forceps, vacuum extraction, and cesarean birth are examples.
- Hemorrhagic (hypovolemic) shock is an emergency in which sufficient blood does not reach vital organs in the mother or newborn; death may ensue.
- The basic purpose of a cesarean delivery is to preserve the life and health of the woman and her fetus.
- Infection control measures are essential to protect the mother and newborn from transmission of infectious organisms.

■ Teaching–Learning Strategies

CLASSROOM

1. Ask the students to define the following terms:

abortion
forceps
placenta previa
abruptio placenta
gestational diabetes
polyhydramnios
hydatidiform mole
amniocentesis
preeclampsia
hematoma
choriocarcinoma
cystitis
preterm labor

hydramnios
dystocia
puerperal
hyperemesis
eclampsia
vacuum extraction
induction
ectopic
version
mastitis
RH sensitization
ABO incompatibility
ultrasonic scanning

Write the students' responses on the chalkboard or on an overhead transparency.

2. Briefly discuss the various types of abortions. Ask the students to define habitual abortion and the procedure used to treat this condition.

3. Review the nursing care for clients hospitalized with pregnancy-induced hypertension and prevention of eclampsia.

4. Outline the effects of diabetes mellitus, cardiac disorders, and chemical dependency in a pregnant client.

5. Before class, on an overhead transparency, write *abruptio placenta* and *placenta previa*. Ask students during class to differentiate these two conditions. Briefly review diagnostic testing of pregnant clients.

6. Briefly review complications of labor and delivery (e.g., premature rupture of the membranes). Ask students to outline nursing care for clients with these complications.

CLINICAL

1. Assign students in the clinical setting to work with a nurse who is caring for a client who is considered high risk. Ask students to write their observations in a short report and share their observations with the larger class.

2. Assign pairs of students to a "high-risk" maternity clinic. Ask the students to interview one of the clients and ask how the client's high-risk pregnancy is affecting her life and family. Ask the students to share their findings with the larger group.

3. Assign a small group of students to observe a cesarean section that is scheduled because the client is in a "high-risk" category. Ask the students to share their observations with the larger group.

4. Assign a small group of students to a hospital or clinic that performs antepartal diagnostic testing (e.g., nonstress tests or ultrasound). Ask the students to share their observations with the larger group.

CHAPTER 68

The High-Risk Newborn

LEARNING OBJECTIVES

1. Define the term *high-risk newborn*.

2. Define and differentiate between the following: AGA, SGA, LGA, LBW, VLBW, RDS, ROP, and macrosomia.

3. Compare and contrast at least three nursing considerations for the care of a preterm infant and a postterm infant.

4. Define and discuss at least three nursing considerations for each of the following: meconium or amniotic fluid aspiration, cyanosis, physiologic jaundice, hyperbilirubinemia, phototherapy, dehydration, NEC, and hypoglycemia.

5. Define and differentiate between Rh sensitization, erythroblastosis fetalis, and ABO incompatibility. State at least three nursing interventions for these hemolytic disorders.

6. State the causes of the following types of birth injuries: fractures, intracranial hemorrhage, brachial plexus injury, and facial paralysis. Discuss at least two nursing interventions for each injury.

7. Define and differentiate between congenital disorders, genetic disorders, and teratogenic disorders.

8. Define the following musculoskeletal disorders: talipes, congenital dislocated hip, polydactylism, and syndactylism. State at least two nursing interventions for each disorder.

9. Describe the following nervous system disorders: hydrocephalus, spina bifida, Down syndrome, anencephaly, and microcephaly. State at least two nursing interventions for each disorder.

10. Define the following cardiovascular disorders: patent ductus arteriosus, ASD, VSD, tetralogy of Fallot, and coarctation of the aorta, and state at least two nursing interventions for each disorder.

11. Define the respiratory disorder choanal atresia and state two appropriate nursing interventions.

12. Define the following gastrointestinal disorders: cleft lip, cleft palate, esophageal atresia, tracheoesophageal fistula, pyloric stenosis, imperforate anus, PKU, galactosemia, exstrophy of the bladder, hypospadias, and epispadias. List at least two nursing interventions for each disorder.

13. Identify the common infections (TORCH) that can adversely affect the fetus. State at least two nursing interventions for each infection.

14. Define and discuss at least three nursing considerations for FAS.

15. Identify at least three consequences to the fetus if the mother has a chemical dependency on alcohol, cocaine, heroin, or marijuana.

NEW TERMINOLOGY

ABO incompatibility	imperforate anus
anencephaly	macrosomia
choanal atresia	microcephaly
cleft lip	phototherapy
cleft palate	physiologic jaundice
congenital	polydactylism
epispadias	postterm
erythroblastosis fetalis	preterm
esophageal atresia	pyloric stenosis
exstrophy	Rh sensitization
galactosemia	spina bifida
high-risk newborn	syndactylism
hydrocephalus	talipes
hyperbilirubinemia	thrush
hypospadias	toxoplasmosis

Acronyms

AGA	PKU
ASD	RDS
CMV	ROP
CSF	SGA
FAS	SIDS
LBW	TORCH
LGA	VLBW
NEC	VSD

KEY POINTS

- High-risk newborns have special problems related to maturity, hemolytic conditions, birth injuries, alterations in structure or function, infections, and chemical dependency.
- Classification of newborns according to size and gestational age will direct their plan of care.
- The nurse's main contribution to the newborn's welfare begins with early observations, accurate documentation, and prompt reporting of abnormal signs.
- Interpreting data, making decisions, and providing therapy are crucial nursing skills when caring for high-risk newborns.
- Nursing care for the preterm infant involves taking into consideration the immaturity of the infant.
- Large-for-gestational age infants have special problems, including hypoglycemia, respiratory disorders, and injuries such as fractures of the clavicle and skull.
- A small number of birth injuries occur despite competent obstetric care.
- Common disorders occur in the various body systems and carry special nursing care considerations.
- The newborn may acquire an infection while in the uterus, during birth, during resuscitation, or while in the nursery.
- Infections and sexually transmitted diseases acquired by the newborn can be life threatening or have long-term sequelae.
- Nurses often are the first to observe signs of drug dependency in newborns.
- The onset of signs and symptoms in newborns experiencing withdrawal vary depending on the drug the mother used.

■ Teaching–Learning Strategies

CLASSROOM

1. Ask students to define the following terms:

anencephaly	esophageal atresia
genetic	phototherapy
pyloric stenosis	teratogenic
atelectasis	galactosemia
hydrocephalus	thrush
RDS	toxoplasmosis
congenital	physiologic jaundice
hypospadias	meconium aspiration
cytomegalovirus	syndrome
microcephaly	necrotizing enterocolitis
spina bifida	exstrophy of the bladder
epispadias	

Write the students' responses on the chalkboard or on an overhead transparency.

2. Briefly review classification of high-risk newborns. Ask students to differentiate between small-for-gestational age, large-for-gestational age, post-term and preterm neonates. Write the students' responses on the chalkboard or on an overhead transparency.

3. Briefly review nursing care of the preterm newborn. Invite a nurse who is employed in a nursery for high-risk newborns to speak to the class about caring for preterm newborns. After the presentation, open the class for questions and discussion.

4. Before class, on 3 × 5 index cards, write a potential complication (e.g., meconium aspiration syndrome), a birth injury (e.g., brachial plexus palsy), or a congenital defect (e.g., exstrophy of the bladder) on each card. During the class, assign students to one or more of the cards while working in pairs. Ask students to identify the condition and treatment/nursing care required for each condition.

5. Briefly discuss the symptoms, care, and treatment of chemically dependent newborns.

6. Ask a representative from the March of Dimes to visit the class and present the topic of "prevention of birth defects." After the presentation, open the class for questions and discussion.

CLINICAL

1. Assign students in pairs to observe in a special care or high-risk nursery. Ask students to focus on one infant in the nursery and write a brief report. Ask students to share their observations with the larger group.

2. Invite a mother who has given birth to a preterm newborn to visit the clinical group (or class) and present her experience with a preterm newborn. After the presentation, open the class for discussion and questions.

3. Assign a small group of students to a pediatric infant unit that cares for newborns with birth injuries or congenital anomalies. Ask the students to observe a nurse caring for these children. Ask students to share their observations with the larger group.

4. Ask students in pairs to design a poster that focuses on prevention of preterm labor or birth defects. Ask the students to share their posters with the larger class. Ask a prenatal clinic if the clinic would like to use the students' posters.

5. Before the clinical experience, ask the students to learn about local community resources for pregnant clients who are chemically dependent. Ask students to share their findings with the larger class.

CHAPTER 69

Sexuality, Fertility, and Sexually Transmitted Diseases

LEARNING OBJECTIVES

1. Define and discuss the concepts of sexuality, sexual orientation, heterosexuality, homosexuality, bisexuality, and asexuality.

2. Identify at least four nursing considerations for the care of an individual who has been raped.

3. State four causes of sexual dysfunction in men and women. Describe at least two medical and surgical interventions for these disorders.

4. Discuss four nursing interventions for male and female infertility. Identify two diagnostic procedures and two forms of treatment for infertility.

5. Define and discuss the following contraception methods: abstinence, withdrawal, BCPs, emergency contraception, Depo-Provera, Norplant system, Lunelle, IUDs, and mechanical and chemical barrier methods.

6. Discuss at least four aspects of client teaching related to sterilization by vasectomy.

7. Discuss four aspects of client teaching related to sterilization by tubal ligation.

8. Differentiate and discuss at least four aspects of client teaching related to the following types of sexually transmitted diseases (STDs): HIV/AIDS, chlamydia, gonorrhea, syphilis, herpes simplex virus (HSV), cytomegalovirus (CMV), human papilloma virus (HPV), chancroid, candidiasis, trichomoniasis, bacterial vaginosis, and pediculosis.

9. Identify the signs and symptoms, diagnostic methods, and treatments for each of the STDs listed above.

10. In the skills lab, prepare a client (mannequin) for the first pelvic examination. Obtain the equipment and assist the healthcare practitioner in obtaining a Pap smear, KOTT slide, and a VDRL.

NEW TERMINOLOGY

artificial insemination	homosexual
asexual	impotence
bacterial vaginosis	infertility
bisexual	lesbian
candidiasis	orgasm
chancre	pediculosis pubis
chancroid	priapism
chlamydia	rape
coitus interruptus	sexual dysfunction
condom	sexual orientation
contraception	sexuality
dyspareunia	sterility
gay	trichomoniasis
genital herpes	tubal ligation
gonorrhea	vaginismus
heterosexual	vasectomy

KEY POINTS

- Human sexuality involves the whole body, mind, and spirit. It is at the core of each individual's personality.
- Sexual assault is a crime of violence. Victims need support, encouragement, and treatment to aid them in dealing with the aftermath.
- Sexual dysfunction is a person's inability to enjoy or engage in sexual activity for any reason.
- Infertility can be caused by male or female factors. Common factors include decreased sperm production, ovulation disorders, tubal obstruction, and endometriosis.
- Contraception is an important consideration for individuals during various stages of their fertile years. Counseling in this area must be nonjudgmental and geared to meet the needs and preferences of the individual.
- Sexually transmitted diseases have the potential to cause sterility and, in some cases, death.

■ Teaching–Learning Strategies

CLASSROOM

1. Ask students to define the following terms:

asexual	vaginismus
impotence	gay
fertility	vasectomy
sexuality	heterosexual
bisexual	pediculosis pubis
sterility	priapism
contraception	homosexual
orgasm	sexual dysfunction
lesbian	mechanical barriers
tubal ligation	chemical barriers
dyspareunia	

   Write the students' responses on the chalkboard or on an overhead transparency.

2. Ask students to list various causes of male and female infertility. Briefly discuss methods to treat infertility.

3. Invite a nurse who is employed in a family planning or fertility clinic to present the role of the nurse in caring for clients desiring contraception or fertility treatments. After the presentation, open the class for questions and discussion.

4. Divide the class into pairs. Assign each pair of students a particular contraception method. Ask students to outline advantages and disadvantages, along with danger signs (if any). Ask the pairs of students to share their findings with the larger class.

5. Briefly discuss the sexually transmitted diseases of gonorrhea, syphilis, herpes simplex 2, chlamydia, genital warts, lice, HIV, and cytomegalovirus.

CLINICAL

1. Assign a small group of students to visit a family planning or Planned Parenthood clinic. Ask the students to observe a nurse in the setting and interview the nurse about the type of services provided by the clinic. Ask the students to share their observations during clinical conference.

2. Assign a small group of students to visit a fertility clinic. Ask the students to observe a nurse in the setting and interview the nurse about the type of services provided by the clinic. Ask the students to share their observations during clinical conference.

3. Assign a small group of students to an outpatient clinic that treats sexually transmitted diseases. Ask the students to observe a nurse in the clinic. Ask the students to share their observations during clinical conference.

4. Ask students in pairs to design a poster related to the topic of contraception. Ask students to share their posters with the larger group. Offer to donate the students' posters to a family planning clinic.

SUGGESTED RESOURCES: VIDEOTAPES

Contraception: Know your options for men and women. (1993). [30 minutes]. (Available from Nimco, Inc., P.O. Box 9, 102 Highway 81 North, Calhoun, KY 42327; #PPI-863-V52)

Epidural analgesia. (1992). [31 minutes]. (Available from Lippincott Williams & Wilkins, 530 Walnut Street, Philadelphia, PA 19106; ISBN 0-397-48055-5)

Fetal alcohol syndrome: A life sentence. [24 minutes]. (Available from Films for the Humanities and Sciences, P. O. Box 2053, Princeton, NJ 08543-2053)

Fetal alcohol syndrome and other drug use during pregnancy. [19 minutes]. (Available from Films for the Humanities and Sciences, P. O. Box 2053, Princeton, NJ 08543-2053)

Gestational age assessment. (1992). [27 minutes]. (Available from Lippincott Williams & Wilkins, 530 Walnut Street, Philadelphia, PA 19106; ISBN 0-397-48055-5)

Maternal newborn nursing. (1996). [CAI]. (Available from Lippincott Williams & Wilkins, 530 Walnut Street, Philadelphia, PA 19106; ISBN 0-397-55306-4)

Physical assessment of the normal newborn (2nd ed.). (1992). [27 minutes]. (Available from Lippincott Williams & Wilkins, 530 Walnut Street, Philadelphia, PA 19106; ISBN 0-397-56782-0)

Planning and conception. (1994). [27 minutes] (Available from Nimco, Inc., P.O. Box 9, 102 Highway 81 North, Calhoun, KY 42327; #NIM-SM-HAB1-V7)

Prenatal care. (1994). [23 minutes]. (Available from Nimco, Inc., P.O. Box 9, 102 Highway 81 North, Calhoun, KY 42327; #NIM-SM-HAB3-V7)

Teen dads' point of view. [40 minutes]. (Available from Films for the Humanities and Sciences, P.O. Box 2053, Princeton, NJ 08543-2053)

The father factor: Paternally caused infertility. [53 minutes]. (Available from Films for the Humanities and Sciences, P.O. Box 2053, Princeton, NJ 08543-2053)

Unborn addicts. [50 minutes]. (Available from Films for the Humanities and Sciences, P.O. Box 2053, Princeton, NJ 08543-2053)

CHAPTER 70

Fundamentals of Pediatric Nursing

LEARNING OBJECTIVES

1. Explain the concepts of "prevention" and "health maintenance" as they pertain to children.

2. State at least six immunizations provided to children. Identify at least three nursing considerations related to immunizations.

3. Discuss at least five specific nursing observations needed for care of an infant, toddler, preschooler, school-age child, and adolescent.

4. Discuss conversations that may occur between a nurse and a child during a hospital admission.

5. Define and differentiate the stages of separation anxiety.

6. State the normal limits of pulse, respiration, temperature, blood pressure, height, and weight for infants and children of different ages.

7. Identify at least five concerns related to pediatric safety during a hospital admission.

8. List four types of pediatric restraints. State at least three nursing concerns regarding pediatric restraints.

9. In the skills lab, demonstrate the application of a urine collection device on an infant. State at least three nursing concerns for this procedure.

10. Describe the steps involved in bathing an infant. Identify at least three nursing concerns for this procedure.

11. Define and differentiate between the following: oxygen mask, mist tent, and Oxy-Hood. State at least three nursing concerns for each.

12. Identify at least two reasons for performing the following: venipuncture, heel stick, and lumbar puncture. State at least three nursing concerns for each procedure.

13. Differentiate and discuss the treatments for fever lower than 102° F (38.8° C) and higher than 102° F (38.8° C). State at least three nursing concerns for each.

14. State at least three nursing concerns when administering PO and IM medications to an infant, a toddler, a preschool child, and a school-age child.

15. State at least eight nursing concerns for a child before and after a surgical procedure.

16. Identify at least five concepts that need to be discussed with the caretakers of a child who is scheduled to undergo a surgical procedure.

NEW TERMINOLOGY

circumoral cyanosis
Denver Developmental Screening Test
health maintenance
health supervision
immunization
pediatrician
pediatrics

KEY POINTS

- Basic care in pediatrics is similar to the care for adults, but some procedures need modifications.
- Pediatrics requires knowledge of developmental milestones; this knowledge helps you determine developmental delays.
- Children may need assistance to meet basic needs simply because of their age.
- Teaching family caregivers is vital because most pediatric care is given at home.
- Very young children are especially susceptible to communicable diseases.
- Maintenance of pediatric safety is vital.
- Vital signs vary according to a person's size and age.
- Children's respiratory tracts are small and susceptible to infection.
- Play is children's work and their means of communication.

- Administration of medications to children involves precise calculation; it usually is based on body weight in kilograms (kg).

▪ Teaching–Learning Strategies

CLASSROOM

1. Review the table for immunizations and the recommended schedule with the students. Ask students what nursing actions can be taken to have more children properly immunized.

2. Divide students into pairs. Ask students to identify methods for calming and assessing children of various age groups. Review general guidelines of caring for pediatric clients.

3. During the class, ask students to compare and contrast the differences of various procedures (e.g., obtaining vital signs) for adults versus children.

4. During the class, ask students to identify ways to keep children safe. Write the student responses on the chalkboard or on an overhead transparency. Include a discussion of pediatric restraints.

5. Review guidelines for administering medications to pediatric clients. Ask students to share their own experiences with medications given to them as children.

6. Ask students to identify guidelines for preoperative and postoperative care for pediatric clients. Write the students' responses on the chalkboard or on an overhead transparency.

CLINICAL

1. In the learning laboratory, show child-sized models and various equipment used for examinations of children. Allow the students an opportunity to handle the equipment. Ask two students to volunteer to role play a situation in which a mother brings a sick child to a clinic. After the role-playing situation, open the class for discussion and questions.

2. Assign students to a pediatric clinic. Ask the students to observe a nurse employed by the clinic. Ask the students to share their observations with the larger class.

3. Assign students to a pediatric inpatient setting. Pair the students with a nurse employed by the unit and ask the student to assist the nurse throughout the clinical days. Ask the students to share their experiences with the group during clinical conference. Discuss how pediatric procedures differ from those of adults.

4. Assign pairs of students to a daycare center or preschool. Ask the students to compare well children with children who are ill. Ask the students to write a brief report (one to two pages) and present their observations in clinical conference.

CHAPTER 71

Care of the Infant, Toddler, or Preschooler

LEARNING OBJECTIVES

1. Compare and contrast the symptoms, treatment, and immunizations for the following preventable communicable diseases: diphtheria, tetanus, pertussis, rubeola, mumps, rubella, varicella, and poliomyelitis. State three nursing considerations for each disease.

2. Compare and contrast the symptoms of streptococcal infections and roseola. Identify at least three nursing considerations for scarlet fever, "strep throat," and rheumatic fever.

3. Compare and contrast the treatment and control of common parasitic infections in children, including scabies, lice, pinworms, giardiasis, roundworms, and hookworms. Identify at least three family teaching concerns for each.

4. Discuss at least three nursing considerations for each of the following common injuries: fractures, lacerations, cuts, puncture wounds, foreign objects, and animal bites.

5. Identify at least two methods of prevention and treatment for the following: burns, poisoning, suffocation, and drowning.

6. Discuss therapeutic communication skills to the parents of a child who died of SIDS.

7. Identify at least five potential clues to neglect, physical abuse, and sexual abuse. Discuss the nurse's role and responsibility related to these conditions.

8. Describe the physical and/or psychological causes of FTT. State at least three nursing considerations related to FTT.

9. Define and discuss at least three nursing implications for the following skin disorders: nevi, rash, and eczema.

10. Define and discuss at least three nursing implications to the following musculoskeletal disorders: dysplasia, talipes, and torticollis.

11. Define and discuss at least three nursing implications for the following neurologic disorders: Reye's syndrome, meningitis, spina bifida, hydrocephalus, microcephaly, febrile seizures, and breath-holding spells.

12. Define and discuss at least three nursing considerations for the following disorders: marasmus, biliary atresia, celiac disease, and PKU.

13. Define and discuss at least three nursing considerations for strabismus, amblyopia, and cataracts in children.

14. Define and discuss at least three nursing considerations related to otitis media, epistaxis, tonsillitis, cleft lip and cleft palate, and baby bottle syndrome.

15. Differentiate and state at least three nursing considerations for the following cardiovascular disorders: ASD/VSD, PDA, TGV, TOF, COA, stenosis, and tricuspid atresia.

16. Differentiate and state at least three nursing considerations for Kawasaki disease, iron deficiency anemia, sickle cell anemia, ITP, and hemophilia.

17. Define and differentiate between the ALL and AML. State at least three nursing considerations for each type of leukemia.

18. Differentiate and state at least three nursing considerations for the following respiratory disorders: URIs, pneumonia, croup, epiglottitis, asthma, bronchiolitis, and cystic fibrosis.

19. Define and state at least three nursing considerations for the following gastrointestinal disorders: pyloric stenosis,

Meckel's diverticulum, intussusception, and megacolon.

20. Identify the types of hernias commonly seen in children. State three pre- and postoperative nursing considerations for hernias.

21. Discuss at least three nursing considerations related to possible electrolyte disturbances and dehydration related to diarrhea in children.

22. Discuss the physical and psychological factors related to encopresis and lactose intolerance.

23. Define and state at least three nursing considerations for the following urinary system disorders: enuresis, HUS, urinary obstruction, UTIs, pyelonephritis, glomerulonephritis, nephrotic syndrome, Wilms' tumor, hypospadias, and epispadias.

24. Define and state at least three nursing considerations for the following reproductive disorders: ambiguous genitalia, cryptorchidism, and hydrocele.

25. Demonstrate a parent–child teaching session related to the nutritional concerns of childhood.

NEW TERMINOLOGY

amblyopia	hernia
asthma	Herpes zoster
biliary atresia	Hirschsprung's disease
bronchiolitis	Hodgkin's disease
celiac disease	hydrocele
cleft lip	hydrocephalus
cleft palate	hypospadia
colic	intussusception
collagen diseases	Kawasaki disease
cryptorchidism	Koplik's spots
cystic fibrosis	Kwashiorkor
diphtheria	lactose intolerance
dysplasia	leukemia
eczema	marasmus
encephalitis	Meckel's diverticulum
encephalocele	megacolon
encopresis	meningitis
enuresis	meningocele
epiglottis	meningomyelocele
epispadias	microcephalic
epistaxis	Mongolian spots
giardiasis	mumps
glomerulonephritis	nephritic syndrome
hemangioma	nevus
hemophilia	otitis media

pediculosis	roundworm
pertussis	rubella
pinworms	rubeola
plumbism	spina bifida
pneumonia	status asthmaticus
pyelonephritis	strabismus
Reye's syndrome	streptococcal "strep" throat
rickets	tetanus
roseola	torticollis

KEY POINTS

- Many childhood communicable diseases can be prevented through immunization.
- Accidents are the number one cause of death in children older than 1 year of age.
- Lack of supervision exists in more than 90% of all near-drowning events.
- SIDS is the sudden, unexplained death of an apparently healthy child.
- The young child depends on others to meet basic needs. When family caregivers do not meet these needs, it is considered child neglect.
- Meningomyelocele, the most serious form of spina bifida, may cause paralysis or other disorders.
- Family caregivers of a child born with facial defects need emotional support and understanding.
- Children with celiac disease must avoid dietary intake of food containing gluten.
- Structural defects of the heart result in abnormal shunting of oxygenated and deoxygenated blood.
- Cystic fibrosis is an autosomal recessive disease of the exocrine glands resulting in serious damage to the lungs, pancreas, and liver.
- Illness of the GI tract places the young child at high risk for fluid and electrolyte imbalance or dehydration.

■ Teaching–Learning Strategies

CLASSROOM

1. Before class, use 3 5 index cards to write the common childhood communicable diseases (e.g., whooping cough). During the class, assign each student pair an index card. Ask the students to identify the disease, its transmission, treatment, and possible complications. Ask the students to share their findings with the larger class.

2. Briefly discuss different types of trauma, such as burns or fractures, that occur in infants, toddlers, or preschoolers. Ask students to share their own experiences.

3. Show the videotape(s) *Child Physical Abuse* (26 minutes) and *Child Sexual Abuse* (26 minutes; both available from Films for the Humanities and Sciences, P.O. Box 2053, Princeton, NJ 08543-2053; 800-257-5126). After viewing the videotapes, open the class for discussion and questions.

4. Before class, on 3 × 5 index cards, write various conditions that affect different body systems (e.g., musculoskeletal: clubfoot). During the class, assign students in pairs to identify the disorder, its causes, treatment, and potential long-term effects.

5. Invite a pediatric nurse who is employed in a specialized area (e.g., cardiovascular, cancer, GI) to visit the class and discuss nursing care of children with these disorders. After the presentation, open the class for discussion and questions.

6. Invite a person who is involved with the Compassionate Friends organization to present their work with families who have had children who have died. After the presentation, open the class for discussion and questions.

CLINICAL

1. Assign students to a pediatric inpatient unit that cares for infants, toddlers, and preschoolers. Pair the students with a nurse employed on the unit and ask the students to assist the nurse throughout the clinical day. After the experience, ask the students to share their observations in clinical conference.

2. Assign a small group of students to observe during a pediatric surgery. After the experience, ask the students to share their observations in clinical conference.

3. Assign a group of students to a well-baby clinic that performs immunizations. Ask the students to observe and assist the staff in the clinic. After the experience, ask the students to share their observations in clinical conference.

4. Ask students to interview a pediatric nurse about her experiences with children who are dying. Ask the students to write a one- to two-page report and share their interviews during clinical conference.

5. Ask students to design a nursing care plan for an infant, toddler, or preschooler with a specific medical disorder, such as Hirschsprung's disease or celiac disease. Ask the students to share their written care plans with the larger class.

CHAPTER 72

Care of the School-Age Child or Adolescent

LEARNING OBJECTIVES

1. Compare and contrast the symptoms and treatment of mononucleosis, Lyme disease, and encephalitis. State three nursing considerations for each infection.

2. Define and discuss at least three nursing implications of the following skin disorders: acne vulgaris, impetigo contagiosa, and tinea pedis.

3. Define and discuss at least three nursing implications of the following musculoskeletal disorders: lordosis, kyphosis, scoliosis, juvenile rheumatoid arthritis, Legg-Calvé-Perthes disease, dental malocclusion, and malignant bone tumors.

4. Compare and contrast at least three nursing implications for diabetes mellitus type 1 and diabetes mellitus type 2.

5. Define and discuss at least three nursing implications of retinitis pigmentosa and juvenile glaucoma.

6. Define and discuss at least three nursing implications of IBD and appendicitis.

7. Define and discuss at least three nursing implications of mittelschmerz and dysmenorrhea.

8. Present a therapeutic teaching session for a family with an adolescent who has concerns about sexual development.

9. Present a therapeutic teaching session for an adolescent with a known or suspected sexually transmitted disease.

10. Define and discuss at least three nursing implications of narcolepsy, hypersomnia, nightmares, somnambulism, night terrors, somniloquism, and insomnia.

11. Identify and differentiate between anorexia nervosa and bulimia nervosa. State three nursing considerations for each condition.

12. Present a therapeutic teaching session to the parents of a child who is obese.

13. Define and discuss at least three nursing implications for enuresis and encopresis.

14. Identify at least three physical and psychological causes of behavioral disorders such as breaking the law and fear of school.

15. Identify at least five nutritional concerns for a school-age child. State at least two nursing considerations for each concern.

NEW TERMINOLOGY

acne vulgaris	Lyme disease
anorexia nervosa	malocclusion
bulimia nervosa	mittelschmerz
cataplexy	mononucleosis
chronic ulcerative colitis	narcolepsy
dermabrasion	orthodontia
dysmenorrhea	polydipsia
encephalitis	polyphagia
hypersomnia	polyuria
impetigo contagiosa	retinitis pigmentosa
insomnia	scoliosis
kyphosis	somnambulism
lordosis	somniloquism

KEY POINTS

- Hormonal changes occurring in the older child result in certain disorders, including acne vulgaris, menstrual difficulties, and emotional disorders.
- School-age children and adolescents often place high importance on their physical appearance and peer acceptance. These factors affect adjustment to many illnesses and disorders.

- The most important aspect of treatment of Legg-Calvé-Perthes disease is maintaining the affected extremity as nonweight-bearing.
- Anorexia nervosa and bulimia, although related to nutrition, are psychological disorders requiring long-term treatment.

■ Teaching–Learning Strategies

CLASSROOM

1. Ask students to define the following terms or abbreviations:

acne	dermabrasion
insomnia	mittelschmerz
polydipsia	sebum
anorexia nervosa	dysmenorrhea
kyphosis	narcolepsy
polyphagia	somnambulism
bulimia	hypersomnia
lordosis	orthodontia
polyuria	somniloquism
cataplexy	glaucoma
malocclusion	STDs
scoliosis	night terrors

Write the students' responses on the chalkboard or on an overhead transparency.

2. Before class, on 3 × 5 index cards, write various conditions that affect different body systems (e.g., juvenile rheumatoid arthritis). During the class, assign students in pairs to identify the disorder, its causes, treatment, and potential long-term effects.

3. Before class, ask student pairs to design an age-specific (e.g., adolescent) poster related to a specific medical disorder affecting this age group. During the class, ask students to present their posters to the class.

4. Invite a nurse who cares for children of this age group in a hospital setting to present the topic of caring for this particular age group. After the presentation, open the class for questions and discussion.

5. Before class, ask the students to review a variety of lay magazines and ask the students to observe the depictions of female models in the advertisements (such models typically are very thin). Ask the students to share their observations with the larger class. Discuss cultural differences about self-perception, particularly with females.

6. Invite a nurse who cares for clients with anorexia nervosa or bulimia to address the class on the topic of eating disorders. After the presentation, open the class for questions and discussion.

CLINICAL

1. Assign students to an inpatient pediatric unit that cares for school-age children or adolescents. Ask the students to assist a staff nurse on the unit for the clinical day. Ask the students to share their experiences during clinical conference.

2. Ask students to design a nursing care plan for a school-age child or adolescent with a specific medical disorder, such as impetigo contagiosa. Ask the students to share their written care plans with the larger class.

3. Assign a small group of students to a prenatal clinic that cares for adolescents who are pregnant. Ask the students to interview one of the clients and ask her about the pregnancy, plans for the baby, and so forth. Ask the students to share their observations with the larger class.

4. Assign a small group of students to an outpatient clinic that cares for school-age or adolescent clients. Ask the students to assist a staff nurse for the clinical day. Ask the students to share their observations with the larger class.

ADDITIONAL RESOURCES

Brosnan, C. A., Upchurch, S., & Schreiner, B. (2001). Type 2 diabetes in children and adolescents: An emerging disease. *Journal of Pediatric Health Care, 15*(4), 187–193.

Dowell, D. L. (1988). Effects of television on children: A review of the literature and recommendations for nurse practitioners. *The American Journal for Nurse Practitioners, 2*(10), 31–37.

Moran, R. (1999). Rebels with a cause: When adolescents won't follow medical advise. *American Journal of Nursing, 98*(12), 26–30.

Ruiz, E. K. (2001). Type 2 diabetes in children. *RN, 64*(10), 44–48.

Stone, K., Paul, B., & Hyatt, D. (2000). Hypercholesterolemia in children. *The American Journal for Nurse Practitioners, 4*(4), 25–31.

Wahl, R. (1999). Nutrition in the adolescent. *Pediatric Annals, 28*(2), 107–111.

CHAPTER 73

The Child or Adolescent With Special Needs

LEARNING OBJECTIVES

1. Define and differentiate between genetic and acquired congenital disorders. State at least three nursing considerations related to these disorders.

2. Identify at least five characteristic signs and symptoms of FAS. Discuss at least four nursing considerations related to maternal alcohol consumption.

3. Identify at least five characteristic signs and symptoms of neonatal abstinence syndrome. Discuss at least four nursing considerations related to prevention and treatment of this syndrome.

4. Identify at least five characteristic signs and symptoms of pediatric HIV/AIDS. Discuss at least four nursing considerations related to prenatal, perinatal, and postnatal care of a woman with HIV.

5. Identify at least four criticisms of standard IQ tests.

6. Define and differentiate between the following levels of mental impairment: borderline, mild, moderate, severe, and profound. State at least two nursing considerations for each level of functioning.

7. Identify at least five characteristics of Down syndrome. Discuss at least four nursing considerations related to the care of an individual with Down syndrome.

8. Define and differentiate between Down syndrome and fragile X syndrome. State at least four nursing considerations related to a child with fragile X syndrome.

9. Discuss at least four effects that developmental and learning disabilities have on the child and the caregivers and family.

10. Identify at least five characteristics of ADHD. Discuss at least four nursing considerations related to the care and upbringing of a child with ADHD.

11. List at least five characteristics of Tourette syndrome. Discuss at least four nursing considerations related to the care and upbringing of a child with TS.

12. Identify at least four characteristics of autism. Discuss at least four nursing considerations related to the care and upbringing of a child with autism.

13. Identify at least four characteristics of plumbism. State at least four major causes of plumbism and four nursing interventions related to the prevention and treatment of plumbism.

14. Identify the main classifications of cerebral palsy. State at least four nursing considerations related to the care and upbringing of a child with CP.

15. Differentiate the causes and treatments of Duchenne muscular dystrophy with Down syndrome and fragile X syndrome.

16. Present a therapeutic teaching session to a new father who has a child with severe sight and hearing loss.

17. Define and differentiate between the characteristics of childhood depression and childhood schizophrenia.

18. Present a nursing conference on an adolescent client who has expressed thoughts of suicide.

19. Discuss at least four nursing concerns related to maternal substance abuse and the potential effects on their children.

20. Identify at least five nursing considerations related to long-term pediatric rehabilitation.

21. Describe how a child's special needs affect the entire family.

NEW TERMINOLOGY

ataxic cerebral palsy	fragile X syndrome
autism	genetics
chelation	Gower's sign
congenital	intellectual or cognitive
developmental disability	impairment
Down syndrome	learning disability
Duchenne muscular	plumbism
dystrophy	schizophrenia
dysfluency	simian line
dyskinetic cerebral palsy	spastic cerebral palsy
dyslexia	suicidal ideation
dysphagia	teratogen
echolalia	trisomy 21

KEY POINTS

- Caregivers of a child with special needs may grieve over the loss of the expected "perfect child."
- A congenital disorder is one that is present at birth. A genetic disorder results from an abnormal gene. A congenitally acquired disorder may result from fetal exposure to teratogens, infections, or trauma.
- Maternal use of alcohol or drugs can result in physical or mental abnormalities in a newborn.
- A common finding in children with learning disabilities is low self-esteem.
- Children with neuromuscular disabilities often have motor, sensory, and developmental delays and feeding problems. A multidisciplinary approach is essential.
- Substance abuse occurs most often in families facing difficulties (e.g., divorce, abuse, chronic alcoholism, financial problems). In many instances, substance abusers have low self-esteem and use drugs to escape reality.
- Families need support and encouragement when managing the care of a child with special needs.

■ Teaching–Learning Strategies

CLASSROOM

1. Ask students to define the following terms or abbreviations:

autism	chromosomes
echolalia	pica
schizophrenia	congenital
chelation	plumbism
genetic disorder	fragile X syndrome
teratogens	spastic
fetal alcohol syndrome	

Write the students' responses on the chalkboard or on an overhead transparency.

2. During the class, ask the students to compare and contrast genetic disorders with acquired disorders. Write the students' responses on the chalkboard or on an overhead transparency.

3. Briefly discuss Down syndrome and list the IQ categories from borderline to profound. Ask students to differentiate Down syndrome from fragile X syndrome.

4. Ask students to identify the criteria for attention deficit hyperactivity disorder. Ask students to identify nursing considerations when caring for children with this disorder.

5. Briefly review autism, chronic lead poisoning, and long-term neuromuscular disorders. Assign students in pairs to develop a nursing care plan for children with these disorders. Ask students to share their care plans with the class. Review the nursing care of children who need rehabilitation or long-term care.

6. Briefly discuss mental illness in children and adolescents. Invite a mental health nurse to visit the class and present the topic of nursing care of children and adolescents with mental illness.

CLINICAL

1. Assign a group of students to a pediatric setting where children with genetic or acquired disorders receive care. Ask the students to share their observations during clinical conference. Ask students in pairs to design a teaching plan or a poster that could be used in a prenatal clinic that focuses on prevention of acquired disorders.

2. Assign a small group of students to an outpatient or an inpatient setting where children with impaired cognitive functioning receive care. Ask students to share their observations during clinical conference.

3. Invite a public health nurse to the clinical conference. Ask the nurse to discuss what efforts are being made in the community to decrease the effects of lead poisoning in children. After the presentation, open the class for discussion and questions.

4. Assign a small group of students to an inpatient mental health setting where children or adolescents receive care. Ask the students to assist the staff nurse in caring for these children. Ask students to share their observations during clinical conference.

5. Assign students to a pediatric rehabilitation center. Ask the students to assist the staff nurse in caring for these children. Ask for two student volunteers to research the costs of long-term care for children or adolescents. Ask students to share their observations during clinical conference.

SUGGESTED RESOURCES: VIDEOTAPES

Assessment of respiratory distress in infants and children. (1988). [20 minutes]. (Available from Lippincott Williams & Wilkins, 530 Walnut Street, Philadelphia, PA 19106)

Caring for sick children. [28 minutes]. (Available from Films for the Humanities and Sciences, P.O. Box 2053, Princeton, NJ 08543-2053; 800-257-5126)

Common childhood illnesses. [45 minutes]. (Available from Films for the Humanities and Sciences, P.O. Box 2053, Princeton, NJ 08543-2053; 800-257-5126)

A head to toe pediatric assessment.(1992). [28 minutes]. (Available from Lippincott Williams & Wilkins, 530 Walnut Street, Philadelphia, PA 19106)

Immunizations. [20 minutes]. (Available from Films for the Humanities and Sciences, P.O. Box 2053, Princeton, NJ 08543-2053; 800-257-5126.)

Pediatric venipuncture. (1994). [14 minutes]. (Available from Lippincott Williams & Wilkins, 530 Walnut Street, Philadelphia, PA 19106)

Raising healthy kids. (Available from Films for the Humanities and Sciences, P.O. Box 2053, Princeton, NJ 08543-2053; 800-257-5126)

ADDITIONAL RESOURCES

Bennett, A. D. (1999). Perinatal substance abuse and the drug-exposed neonate. *Advance for Nurse Practitioners* 7(5), 33–36.

Burke, S. O., Kauffman, E., Harrison, M. B., & Wiskin, N. (1999). Assessment of stressors in families with a child who has a chronic condition. *The American Journal of Maternal Child Nursing, 24*(2), 98–106.

Dumas, D. (1999). A study of self-perception in hyperactive children. *The American Journal of Maternal Child Nursing, 24*(1), 12–19.

Fleitas, J. (2000). When Jack fell down ... Jill came tumbling after: Siblings in the web of illness and disability. *The American Journal of Maternal Child Nursing, 25*(5), 267–273.

Gardner, J. (2000). Living with a child with fetal alcohol syndrome. *The American Journal of Maternal Child Nursing, 25*(5), 252–257.

Jiwanlal, S. S., & Weitzel, C. (2001). The suicide myth. *RN, 64*(1), 33–37.

Johnson, B. S. (2000). Mothers' perceptions of parenting children with disabilities. *The American Journal of Maternal Child Nursing, 25*(3), 127–132.

Kownig, K. (1998). Pervasive development disorders: Diagnosis, intervention, and education. *The American Journal of Nurse Practitioners, 2*(8), 15–28.

Ruppert, R. (1999). The last smoke. *The American Journal of Nursing, 99*(11), 26–32.

Smucker, J. M. (2001). Managed care and children with special health care needs. *Journal of Pediatric Health Care, 15*(1), 3–9.

ViRiper, M., & Cohen, W. I. (2001). Caring for children with Down syndrome and their families. *Journal of Pediatric Health Care, 15*(3), 123–131.

CHAPTER 74

Skin Disorders

LEARNING OBJECTIVES

1. State at least four functions of the integumentary system.

2. Differentiate between the following diagnostic tests: Wood's light examination, Tzanck's smear, tissue biopsy, and scabies scraping.

3. Discuss the two major types of skin grafts and state at least three nursing considerations for care of the skin grafts.

4. Identify at least eight types of skin lesions and give an example of each.

5. State at least four possible nursing diagnoses for a client with a chronic skin disorder.

6. Relate at least three nursing interventions for the care of a client with pruritus.

7. Define and differentiate between the following: urticaria, vitiligo, dermatitis, eczema, and psoriasis. State at least two nursing considerations for each.

8. Define and differentiate between the following: warts, condylomata acuminata, impetigo, and folliculitis. State at least two nursing considerations for each.

9. Define and differentiate between the following: scabies, lice, bedbugs, sebaceous cysts, seborrhea, seborrheic dermatitis, and dandruff. State at least two nursing considerations for each.

10. Identify the four mechanisms that cause burns.

11. Explain how burns are classified according to depth and size.

12. Describe the three phases of recovery in burn therapy, including assessment and treatment of fluid and electrolyte imbalances, respiratory dysfunction, renal changes, infection, and pain.

13. Describe at least four types of dressings and four types of topical medications used when treating burns.

14. Explain the process of debridement and skin grafting to treat burns.

15. Identify at least five complications that occur during burn recovery.

16. Discuss at least four nursing considerations during the rehabilitative stage of burn healing.

17. Identify three common nonmalignant skin lesions.

18. Define and differentiate basal cell carcinoma, squamous cell carcinoma, and malignant melanoma.

19. Discuss at least four interventions that can be used to prevent skin cancer.

NEW TERMINOLOGY

allograft	eschar
angioedema	folliculitis
angioma	furuncle
autograft	heterograft
biopsy	homograft
carbuncle	impetigo
condylomata acuminata	keloid
contracture	neoplasm
cryosurgery	pruritus
cultured epithelial autograft	psoriasis
debridement	scabies
dermatitis	urticaria
dermatology	vitiligo
eczema	warts
electrodesiccation	xenograft

KEY POINTS

- Dermatology is the study of skin diseases.
- The integumentary system, which is comprised of the skin and its accessory organs, protects the body in various ways: it prevents microorganisms from entering the body; keeps the body from losing too much fluid; regulates body temperature, and helps prevent injury to fragile organs.

- Common diagnostic tests used to determine skin disorders are Wood's light examination, Tzanck's smear, tissue biopsy, and scabies scraping.
- A variety of pharmacologic and nonpharmacologic measures are used to treat pruritus.
- Various allergies may cause urticaria and contact dermatitis.
- Chronic skin disorders include vitiligo, dermatitis, and psoriasis.
- Folliculitis and carbuncles are common bacterial skin infections.
- Parasitic skin infestations are scabies, lice, and bedbugs.
- The four types of burns are thermal, electrical, chemical, and radiation.
- The three major phases of recovery in burns are resuscitative, acute, and rehabilitative.
- Extent of burns is determined by a variety of means. Burn depth and percentage of body surface area burned are significant.
- The major types of skin grafts are autografts, allografts, heterografts, and cultured epithelial autografts.
- Moles, angiomas, and keloids are nonmalignant skin tumors.
- Basal cell carcinoma, squamous cell carcinoma, and malignant melanoma are types of skin cancer.

■ Teaching–Learning Strategies

CLASSROOM

1. Ask the students to define the following terms:

allograft	psoriasis
debridement	carbuncle
keloid	biopsy
angioedema	electrodesiccation
dermatitis	contracture folliculitis
neoplasm	warts
malignant	cryosurgery
melanoma	heterograft
autograft	xenograft
eczema	homograft
vitiligo	impetigo
pruritus	condylomata
scabies	acuminata
eschar	

Write the students' responses on the chalkboard or on an overhead transparency.

2. Show the following videotapes related to burns: *Critical Care: Emergency Burn Treatment* (1995; 26 minutes) and *From Victim to Survivor: Managing the Patient With Burns* (1995; 26 minutes; both available from Lippincott Williams & Wilkins, 530 Walnut Street, Philadelphia, PA 19106). After the videotape presentation(s), open the class for questions and discussion.

3. Before class, on 3 × 5 index cards, write various skin disorders, such as scabies. During the class, divide students into pairs and give each pair an index card labeled with a skin disorder. Ask the students to outline a nursing care plan for the client with this disorder. Ask the students to share their nursing care plans with the larger group.

4. Ask a nurse who cares for burn victims to visit the class and present her role in working with these clients. After the presentation, open the class for questions and discussion.

5. Assign students to search the Internet for resources and support groups for clients with skin disorders. Ask the students to share their findings with the larger group.

CLINICAL

1. In the clinical laboratory, assign students in pairs to practice conducting a skin assessment on their partner. Ask students to share their assessments with the larger group.

2. Assign small groups of students to work with a nurse on a burn unit. Ask the students to share their experiences with the larger group.

3. Assign small groups of students to work with a nurse in a dermatology clinic. After the experience, ask the students to share their observations with the larger group.

ADDITIONAL RESOURCES

American Academy of Dermatology, website: *www.aad.org*
American Burn Association, website: *www.ameriburn.org*
Dermatology Foundation, website: *www.dermfnd.org*
National Burn Victim Foundation, website: *www.nbvf.com*
National Institute of Arthritis and Musculoskeletal and Skin Diseases, National Institutes of Health, website: *www.nih.gov/niams*
National Psoriasis Foundation, website: *www.psoriasis.org*
Skin Cancer Foundation, website: *www.skincancer.org*

CHAPTER 75

Disorders in Fluid and Electrolyte Balance

LEARNING OBJECTIVES

1. Define and differentiate between the following fluid compartments: intracellular, extracellular, interstitial, and intravascular.

2. Discuss at least four major nursing responsibilities associated with laboratory tests ordered by a clinician.

3. In a skills lab demonstration, present a client and family teaching session on the importance of fluid and electrolyte balance with emphasis on the types of care that may be needed for the client.

4. Identify at least four possible causes of fluid volume excess and state at least two nursing considerations for each cause.

5. Identify at least four causes of edema and differentiate between the types of edema.

6. State at least two nursing considerations for dependent edema, sacral edema, pitting and nonpitting edema, and pulmonary edema.

7. Identify at least four possible causes of fluid volume deficit and state at least two nursing considerations for each cause.

8. State the normal serum levels for the following electrolytes: sodium, potassium, calcium, magnesium, chloride, and phosphorus.

9. Identify at least four causes of hypernatremia and hyponatremia.

10. Discuss the major symptoms associated with hypernatremia and hyponatremia. State at least three nursing considerations related to these conditions.

11. Identify at least four causes of hyperkalemia and hypokalemia.

12. Discuss the major symptoms associated with hyperkalemia and hypokalemia. State at least three nursing considerations related to these conditions.

13. Identify at least four causes of hypercalcemia and hypocalcemia.

14. Discuss the major symptoms associated with hypercalcemia and hypocalcemia. State at least three nursing considerations related to these conditions.

15. Identify at least four causes of hypermagnesemia and hypomagnesemia.

16. Discuss the major symptoms associated with hypermagnesemia and hypomagnesemia. State at least three nursing considerations related to these conditions.

17. Identify at least four causes of hyperphosphatemia and hypophosphatemia.

18. Discuss the major symptoms associated with hyperphosphatemia and hypophosphatemia. State at least three nursing considerations related to these conditions.

19. Define and differentiate between respiratory and metabolic acidosis. State the importance of chloride, bicarbonate ions, and hydrogen ions.

20. Define and differentiate between respiratory and metabolic alkalosis. State the importance of chloride, bicarbonate ions, and hydrogen ions.

21. Identify at least four nursing considerations related to data collection, assessment, monitoring, and care of a client with acidosis and a client with alkalosis.

NEW TERMINOLOGY

acidosis
alkalosis
anasarca
ascites
dehydration
edema
fluid volume deficit
fluid volume excess
hypercalcemia
hyperchloremia
hyperkalemia
hypernatremia
hyperphosphatemia

hypocalcemia
hypochloremia
hypokalemia
hypomagnesemia
hyponatremia
hypophosphatemia
metabolic acidosis
metabolic alkalosis
overhydration
pitting edema
respiratory acidosis
respiratory alkalosis
turgor

KEY POINTS

- Fluid and electrolyte disturbances are possible in anyone. They are particularly common in ill and hospitalized clients, including those undergoing surgical and diagnostic procedures. The risk of serious disturbances increases in clients at the extremes of the age spectrum.
- Regular nursing care should include assessment of the client's hydration level.
- Edema is a symptom of many disorders but most commonly indicates fluid overload. Edematous skin is friable and prone to breakdown. Good skin care is imperative, as is client positioning.
- Measurement of I&O and daily weights is an important component in the assessment of fluid balance.
- Respiratory acidosis, if not corrected, could lead to the need for mechanical ventilation.
- A simple treatment for respiratory alkalosis, usually caused by hyperventilation, is for clients to breathe into a bag, retaining needed CO_2 in the body.

■ Teaching–Learning Strategies

CLASSROOM

1. Ask the students to define the following terms:

   acidosis
   alkalosis
   dehydration
   fluid volume deficit
   fluid volume excess
   ascites
   metabolic acidosis

   respiratory acidosis
   metabolic alkalosis
   intracellular
   extracellular
   hypokalemia
   hyperkalemia

Write the students' responses on the chalkboard or on an overhead transparency.

2. Ask the students to discuss reasons a client may have a fluid volume excess, edema, or a fluid volume deficit.

3. Before class, using 3×5 cards, write one of the various electrolytes on each card. During the class, assign one electrolyte to each pair of students. Ask the students to describe the functions of the electrolyte, disorders, and comments. Ask the students to share their findings with the larger group.

4. Ask students to compare and contrast the differences between respiratory acidosis, metabolic acidosis, respiratory alkalosis, and metabolic alkalosis. Write the students' responses on the chalkboard or on an overhead transparency.

CLINICAL

1. In the learning laboratory, have the students practice with intravenous solutions and other materials related to intravenous therapies. Ask the students to assess each other in pairs for edema or dehydration. Have the students role play the procedure for calculating I&O.

2. In the clinical setting, assign students to work with a nurse who is caring for a client with fluid volume excess or deficit. After the experience, ask the students to share their observations with the larger group.

3. Before their clinical experience, ask the students to write a nursing care plan for a client with fluid volume excess, fluid volume deficit, acidosis, or alkalosis. Ask the students to share their nursing care plans with the larger group.

4. In the clinical setting, ask the students to locate the institution's chart that depicts commonly used containers and their amounts for calculation of I&O. Ask the students to practice the procedure for I&O on a client in the clinical setting.

CHAPTER 76

Musculoskeletal Disorders

LEARNING OBJECTIVES

1. In relationship to a client with a musculoskeletal disorder, discuss the diagnostic benefits of the following laboratory tests: ESR, CBC, RF, uric acid, CK, calcium, and phosphorus levels.

2. In relationship to a client with a musculoskeletal disorder, discuss the diagnostic benefits of the following procedures: x-ray, arthrogram, myelogram, CT, MRI, bone scan, ultrasound, arthrocentesis, arthroscopy, bone biopsy, and EMG.

3. Identify and discuss at least six components of data collection (assessment) that are obtained for a client with a musculoskeletal disorder. Relate these components to NANDA nursing diagnoses.

4. Identify and discuss at least four major components of nursing care necessary to protect the client from the hazards of immobilization.

5. Identify and discuss at least four common sites of amputation. State the abbreviations for each site.

6. Define and discuss phantom limb pain. State at least three nursing considerations for this condition.

7. Discuss at least six components of nursing care for a client who has a new limb prosthesis.

8. Discuss at least six aspects of nursing care for a client who has been surgically treated for IVD or HNP.

9. State at least three nursing considerations for clients with TMJ, muscular dystrophy, or osteoporosis.

10. Define and differentiate between the following conditions: RA, OA, ankylosing spondylitis, bursitis, tenosynovitis, carpal tunnel syndrome, and lateral epicondylitis. State at least four nursing considerations for each disorder.

11. Define and differentiate between the following conditions: gout, SLE, scleroderma, and rickets or osteomalacia. State at least four nursing considerations for each disorder.

12. Define and differentiate between a strain, a sprain, and a fracture. State at least four nursing care measures for each condition.

13. State the four categories and at least five types of common fractures.

14. Compare and contrast the advantages and disadvantages of a plaster cast versus a synthetic cast.

15. State at least six nursing implications for the care of a client in a cast.

16. Define and differentiate between skin traction and skeletal traction. State at least three nursing considerations for each type of traction.

17. Identify at least three nursing considerations for clients with a halo device or skull tongs.

18. Define and discuss at least three nursing measures for care of clients with the following treatments: external fixation, ORIF, and arthroplasty.

19. Discuss at least four specific nursing measures for a client with a surgical repair of a hip fracture.

20. Identify and discuss at least nine complications of fractures or bone surgery. Identify at least three nursing considerations for each complication.

21. Define and differentiate between primary and metastatic bone tumors.

NEW TERMINOLOGY

acrosclerosis	kyphosis
amputation	myelogram
ankylosis	orthopedics
arthritis	osteomalacia
arthrocentesis	osteomyelitis
arthrogram	prosthesis
arthroplasty	replantation
arthroscopy	rickets
bursitis	sclerodactyly
compartment syndrome	scleroderma
dislocation	scoliosis
electromyogram	sequestration
fasciotomy	skeletal traction
fracture	skin traction
gangrene	spinal stenosis
gout	synovectomy
halo device	tenosynovitis
hyperuricemia	

KEY POINTS

- Tests that diagnose musculoskeletal disorders include blood tests, x-ray, MRI, CT scan, arthrogram, bone scan, ultrasound, arthrocentesis, arthroscopy, biopsy, and electromyogram.
- Careful nursing assessments and knowledge of potential neurovascular complications are essential in orthopedic nursing. Be aware of and try to prevent complications caused by the client's decreased mobility.
- The many different methods of treating orthopedic injuries include casts, splints, internal fixation, external fixation, traction, and surgeries such as arthroscopy, total joint replacement, and lumbar decompression.
- A cast stabilizes and immobilizes fractures. When clients are wearing casts, carefully assess their neurovascular status, provide pain relief, and protect the casts.
- In skin traction, the pull is applied to the skin; in skeletal traction the traction is applied directly to the bones.
- Early treatment of orthopedic complications is necessary to prevent additional injury to the area involved.
- Potential orthopedic complications include compartment syndrome, wound infection, osteomyelitis, hypostatic pneumonia, embolism, deep vein thrombosis, and hemorrhage.
- Treatment of musculoskeletal disorders and diseases can include drug therapy, exercise, surgery, amputation, physical therapy, diet, or resting the affected part.

- Traumatic musculoskeletal injuries, such as sprains, strains, dislocations, and fractures, require different forms of treatment.
- Primary benign bone tumors grow slowly and rarely spread. Metastatic bone tumors originate elsewhere in the body and are associated with a poor prognosis.

■Teaching–Learning Strategies

CLASSROOM

1. Ask the students to define the following terms:

amputation	arthroplasty
dislocation	gout
prosthesis	myelogram
osteomyelitis	sequestration
ankylosis	orthopedics
fasciotomy	bursitis
fixation	tenosynovitis
replantation	carpal tunnel syndrome
arthritis	arthrogram
fracture	rickets
neoplasm	embolism
scleroderma	halo device

Write the students' responses on the chalkboard or on an overhead transparency.

2. Conduct a discussion about the various diagnostic tests used for clients with musculoskeletal disorders. Ask the students to share their personal or clinical experiences with the diagnostic tests.

3. Review types of casts and traction that are used with clients experiencing a musculoskeletal disorder.

4. Ask the students to describe neurovascular assessments that are necessary when caring for a client with a musculoskeletal disorder.

5. Before class, on 3 × 5 index cards write a complication that can result from a musculoskeletal disorder (e.g., osteomyelitis). During the class divide students into pairs and assign one or more of the complications to each pair. Ask the students to describe signs and symptoms of the complication and share their findings with the class. Use the same technique for common and systemic musculoskeletal disorders and have the students formulate a short nursing care plan to share with the class.

6. Show the videotape *Orthopedic Complications and How to Handle Them* (1993; 30 minutes; available from Lippincott Williams & Wilkins, 530 Walnut Street, Philadelphia, PA 19106). After the videotape presentation, open the class for questions and discussion.

CLINICAL

1. In the clinical laboratory, have students practice ambulating clients with aids such as walkers and canes. Role play a situation in which one of the students is a client who has undergone hip replacement surgery and another student is a nurse. Ask the "nurse" to ambulate the "client" for the first time after surgery.

2. In the clinical setting, assign students to work with a nurse who is caring for a client with a musculoskeletal disorder. After the experience, ask the students to share their experiences and their nursing care plans for the client.

3. Assign small groups of students to an operating room setting where musculoskeletal disorders are treated. Ask the students to document the client's disorder, the type of surgery, and the immediate postoperative care. After the observation, ask the students to share their experiences with the larger group.

4. Assign a small group of students to observe in a physical therapy unit or in a diagnostic center that diagnoses musculoskeletal disorders. After the observation, ask the students to share their experiences with the larger group.

ADDITIONAL RESOURCES

Arthritis Foundation, P.O. Box 7669, Atlanta, GA 30357-0669; telephone: 404-872-7100; website: *www.arthritis.org*

March of Dimes Birth Defects Foundation, 1275 Mamaroneck Avenue, White Plains, NY 10605; telephone: 888-MODIMES (888-663-4637); website: *www.modimes.org*

Muscular Dystrophy Association, 3300 East Sunrise Avenue, Tucson, AZ 85718; telephone: 800-572-1717; website: *www.mdausa.org*

National Amputation Foundation, 38-40 Church Street, Malverne, NY 11565; telephone: 516-877-3600; website: *www.nationalamputation.org*

National Association of Orthopaedic Nurses, Inc., East Holly Avenue, Box 56, Pitman, NJ 08071-0056; telephone: 856-256-2310; website: *www.orthopaedicnurse.org*

National Institute of Arthritis and Musculoskeletal and Skin Disorders, National Institutes of Health, Bethesda, MD 20892; telephone: 301-496-4000

National Multiple Sclerosis Society, 733 3rd Avenue, New York, NY 10017; telephone: 800-344-4867 (800-Fight MS); website: *www.nmss.org*

National Osteoporosis Foundation, 1232 22nd Street NW, Washington, DC 20037-1292; telephone: 202-223-2226; website: *www.nof.org*

National Scoliosis Foundation, 5 Cabot Place, Stoughton, MA 02072; telephone: 800-673-6922 (800-NSF-MYBACK); e-mail: *www.nsf@scoliosis.org*

CHAPTER 77

Nervous System Disorders

LEARNING OBJECTIVES

1. State at least three indications for the use of CT, PET, and MRI in a client with a nervous system disorder.

2. Discuss at least four nursing considerations for the care of a client having an MRI and identify at least five circumstances when an MRI is contraindicated.

3. Define and differentiate between the following diagnostic tests: cerebral angiography, cerebral arteriography, myelography, brain scan, electroencephalography, and videotelemetry.

4. Identify at least six indications for a lumbar puncture. State at least three nursing considerations related to an LP.

5. List at least eight NANDA diagnoses that reflect actual or potential concerns related to a nervous system disorder.

6. Differentiate between migraine and cluster headaches. State at least three nursing considerations for each condition.

7. State the main characteristics of at least three types of partial seizures.

8. State the main characteristics of at least six types of general seizures.

9. State at least four nursing implications for seizure disorders, epilepsy, and status epilepticus.

10. Discuss the causes, signs and symptoms, and nursing implications for the following: trigeminal neuralgia, Bell's palsy, and herpes zoster.

11. Differentiate paraplegia from quadriplegia. Discuss at least four differences in nursing care for each condition.

12. Define autonomic dysreflexia and state at least five signs and symptoms of this condition.

13. Discuss the cause, signs and symptoms, therapies, and at least five nursing considerations for the following degenerative disorders: multiple sclerosis, Parkinson's disease, myasthenia gravis, Huntington's disease, and amyotrophic lateral sclerosis.

14. Discuss the cause, signs and symptoms, therapies, and at least five nursing considerations for the following inflammatory disorders: brain abscess, meningitis, encephalitis, Guillain-Barré syndrome, post-polio syndrome, and acute transverse myelitis.

15. Explain at least four causes of increased intracranial pressure.

16. Define and state at least three nursing considerations related to the following disorders: concussion, brain laceration and contusion, skull fractures, and hematoma.

17. Differentiate between herniation of the brain, intracranial hematoma, epidural hematoma, and a subdural hematoma. State at least three nursing considerations for each.

18. State at least three nursing considerations related to care of a client with a brain tumor.

19. Explain the purpose of a craniotomy. Identify at least three pre- and postoperative nursing considerations for a craniotomy.

NEW TERMINOLOGY

ataxia	dysphonia
aura	epilepsy
autonomic dysreflexia	flaccidity
bradykinesia	focal point
cephalalgia	focus
chorea	intracranial pressure
concussion	laceration
contusion	neuralgia
craniotomy	neurology
diplopia	nuchal rigidity
dysphagia	opisthotonos
dysphasia	paraplegia

parkinsonism	seizure
photophobia	shingles
ptosis	subdural hematoma
quadriplegia	vertigo

KEY POINTS

- Because the nervous system controls the body's movements, disorders in this system may cause unwanted movement or immobility.
- Seizure disorders have different manifestations, ranging from generalized tonic-clonic movements to uncontrolled movements without loss of consciousness.
- Degenerative disorders of the nervous system may cause difficulties in movement, sensory deficits, or varying degrees of alteration in mental status.
- Inflammatory disorders of the nervous system can quickly become life threatening.
- Brain and spinal cord injuries can result in a range of physical and mental deficits, including paralysis.
- Increased intracranial pressure has many causes. It is a significant sign of a brain disorder. One of the first and most important signs of ICP (and other disorders of the brain) is a change in the level of consciousness.
- Most brain tumors are nonmalignant. However, benign tumors cause pressure on the brain and can be fatal. Some resources state that these tumors are malignant by location.

■ Teaching–Learning Strategies

CLASSROOM

1. Ask the students to define the following terms:

ataxia	cephalalgia
epilepsy	subdural hematoma
multiple sclerosis	craniotomy
aura	concussion
seizure	autonomic dysreflexia
intracranial pressure	laceration
bradykinesia	herniation
neuralgia	Bell's palsy
shingles	Huntington's disease
vertigo	myasthenia gravis

Write the students' responses on the chalkboard or on an overhead transparency.

2. Before class, on 3 × 5 index cards, list common nervous system disorders. During the class, assign pairs of students to one disorder and have them formulate a short nursing care plan to share with the class.

3. Ask students to identify symptoms of intracranial pressure. List the students' responses on the chalkboard or on an overhead transparency.

4. Invite a nurse who cares for clients with nervous system disorders or trauma to the class to describe the role of the nurse in caring for these clients. After the presentation, open the class for questions and discussion.

CLINICAL

1. In the clinical setting, assign students in pairs to observe diagnostic testing for clients with nervous system disorders. After the experience, ask the students to share their observations.

2. In the clinical setting, assign students to work with a nurse who is caring for a client with a nervous system disorder. After the experience, ask the students to share their experiences and nursing care plans with the larger group.

3. Assign a small number of students to observe in an operating room setting where surgery is being performed on clients with nervous system disorders. After the experience, ask the students to share their experiences and nursing care plans with the larger group.

4. Ask the students to visit the library or use the Internet to locate one or two articles related to nervous system disorders. Ask the students to share their findings with the larger group.

5. Ask the students to research the local community services available to clients with nervous system disorders. Ask the students to share their findings with the larger group.

ADDITIONAL RESOURCES

ALS Association of America (ALSA), 27001 Agoura Road, Suite 150, Calabasas Hills, CA 91301-5104; telephone: 818-880-9007 or 800-782-4747; fax: 818-880-9006; website: *www.alsa.org/*

American Parkinson's Disease Association, Inc., 1250 Hylan Boulevard, Suite 4B, Staten Island, NY 10305-1946; telephone: 718-981-8001 (Calif: 800-908-2732); fax: 718-981-4399; E-mail: *info@apdaparkinson.org* websites: *www.apdaparkinson.com, www.apdaparkinson.org*

BRAIN, P.O. Box 5801, Bethesda, MD 20824; telephone: 301-496-5751 or 800-352-9424

Epilepsy Foundation of America, 4351 Garden City Drive, Landover, MD 20785-7223; telephone: 800-332-1000; website: *www.efa.org*

Guillain-Barré Foundation International, P.O. Box 262, Wynnewood, PA 19096; telephone: 610-667-0131; website: *www.webmast.com/gbs*

Huntington's Disease Society of America, 158 West 29th Street, 7th floor, New York, NY 10001-5300; telephone: 212-242-1968 or 800-345-HDSA (4372); fax: 212-239-3430; E-mail: *hdsainfo@hdsa.org;* website: *www.hdsa.org*

International Polio Network, 5100 Oakland Avenue, #206, St. Louis, MO 63110-1406; telephone: 314-534-0475

March of Dimes, Birth Defects Foundation, Community Services Department, 1275 Mamaroneck Avenue, White Plains, NY 10605; telephone: 914-428-7100

Myasthenia Gravis Foundation of America, 5841 Cedar Lake Road, Suite 204, Minneapolis, MN 55416; telephone: 800-541-5454 or 952-545-9438; website: *www.myasthenia.org*

National Head Injury Foundation, 333 Turnpike Road, Southborough, MA 01722; telephone: 508-485-9950

National Hydrocephalus Foundation, 12413 Centralis Road, Lakewood, CA 90715-1623; telephone: 562-402-3523; website: *www.nhfonline.org*

National Multiple Sclerosis Society, 733 Third Avenue, New York, NY 10017; telephone: 800-Fight MS (800-344-4867); website: *www.nmss.org*

National Parkinson Foundation, Inc., 1501 NW 9th Avenue, Bob Hope Road, Miami, FL 33136; telephone: 305-547-6666; website: *www.parkinson.org*

National Spinal Cord Injury Association, 5701 Democracy Boulevard, Suite 300-9, Bethesda, MD 20817; telephone: 800-962-9629; website: *www.spinalcord.org*

NIH Neurological Institute, P.O. Box 5801, Bethesda, MD 20824; telephone: 301-496-5751 or 800-352-9424; website: *www.ninds.nih.gov*

Parkinson's Disease Foundation Medical Center, William Black Medical Research Building, 640 West 168th Street, New York, NY 10032; telephone: 212-923-4700

CHAPTER 78

Endocrine Disorders

LEARNING OBJECTIVES

1. Identify the endocrine glands and their hormones.

2. Name the common laboratory tests and radiology procedures performed to evaluate functioning of the pituitary, thyroid, parathyroid, adrenals, and pancreas.

3. Define and differentiate between the four major tests used to test blood glucose levels.

4. Identify at least six NANDA nursing diagnoses that are appropriate for a client with an endocrine disorder of the pituitary, thyroid, parathyroid, and pancreas.

5. Define and differentiate between gigantism and acromegaly and SIADH and diabetes insipidus. State at least three nursing considerations for each.

6. Define and differentiate between Grave's disease, cretinism, and myxedema. State at least three nursing considerations for each.

7. Discuss the known causes of Hashimoto's thyroiditis and simple goiter. State at least three nursing considerations for each.

8. State at least five pre- and postoperative nursing considerations for a client who is undergoing a thyroidectomy.

9. Differentiate between hyperparathyroidism and hypoparathyroidism.

10. Define and differentiate between Cushing's syndrome, primary aldosteronism, and Addison's disease. State at least three nursing considerations for each.

11. State the three main criteria for the diagnosis of diabetes mellitus.

12. Define and differentiate between type 1 and type 2 diabetes mellitus, gestational diabetes, and impaired glucose homeostasis.

13. Discuss the three main criteria of a diabetic regimen.

14. List the three common groups of insulins, stating their onset, peak, and durations of actions.

15. List the four common groups of oral antidiabetic agents and give examples of each.

16. Define and differentiate between hypoglycemia and hyperglycemia as it relates to diabetes. State at least three nursing interventions for each.

17. Define and differentiate between DKA and a nonketotic hyperosmolar state. Identify at least three nursing considerations for each.

18. Define and differentiate between macrovascular and microvascular complications of diabetes giving examples of each.

19. Prepare a teaching plan for a client with diabetes; the plan should cover at least 10 topics of discussion.

20. In the skills lab, demonstrate the use of a blood glucose monitor.

NEW TERMINOLOGY

acromegaly	hypothyroidism
Addison's disease	insulin resistance
cretinism	ketoacidosis
Cushing's syndrome	myxedema
diabetes insipidus	negative feedback system
diabetes mellitus	nephropathy
exophthalmos	neuropathy
giantism	pheochromocytoma
goiter	polydipsia
Graves' disease	polyphagia
hyperglycemia	polyuria
hyperparathyroidism	retinopathy
hyperthyroidism	Somogyi phenomenon
hypoglycemia	thyroidectomy
hypoparathyroidism	

KEY POINTS

- Endocrine glands secrete hormones that influence metabolism, growth, and development.
- Laboratory diagnostic tests for the endocrine system include serum hormone levels, various glucose tests, several urinalysis tests, radiology procedures, and occasionally iodine uptake tests.
- Many endocrine disorders affect growth, development, and appearance.
- The majority of endocrine disorders result from overproduction or underproduction of specific hormones.
- Nursing procedures in the care of a client who has undergone a thyroidectomy include careful monitoring and preparation for emergency care.
- Diabetes mellitus occurs when the pancreas does not make enough insulin or the body becomes resistant to insulin.
- Clients with type 1 diabetes must use insulin as part of their treatment regimen.
- Clients with type 2 diabetes may use oral antidiabetic agents that affect insulin secretion and/or metabolism. Some clients with type 2 diabetes also use insulin.
- Meal planning, exercise, and medications, as needed, are essential components of diabetes management.
- Complications of diabetes affect all aspects of life. Members of the diabetes team work to provide accurate and thorough client teaching and to avoid related complications of the disease.

■ Teaching–Learning Strategies

CLASSROOM

1. Ask the students to define the following terms:

acromegaly	diabetes insipidus
giantism	endocrinologist
hypothyroidism	polyuria
Graves' disease	exophthalmos
Addison's disease	hyperglycemia
Chvostek's sign	insulin
cretinism	Trousseau's sign
goiter	Cushing's syndrome
ketoacidosis	polyphagia

Write the students' responses on the chalkboard or on an overhead transparency.

2. Briefly discuss diagnostic tests, surgical treatments, and signs and symptoms of pituitary or adrenal disorders. Ask students to locate the various endocrine glands.

3. Show the videotape *Diabetes: The Quiet Killer* (26 minutes; available from Films for the Humanities and Sciences, P.O. Box 2053, Princeton, NJ 08543-2053). After the videotape presentation, open the class for questions and discussion.

4. Ask students to compare and contrast hypoglycemia and hyperglycemia. List the signs and symptoms for each on the chalkboard or on an overhead transparency.

CLINICAL

1. In the learning laboratory, have the students divide into pairs to practice blood glucose testing. Students can practice on themselves or on each other.

2. Ask the students to formulate a nursing care plan for clients with an endocrine disorder, such as hypopituitarism. Ask the students to share their care plans in clinical conference.

3. Assign students in a clinical setting to a client who is experiencing an endocrine disorder (e.g., diabetes mellitus.). Ask the students to share their experiences and plan of care for the clients with the larger group.

4. Assign small groups of students to a clinic that cares for clients with endocrine disorders. Ask the students to share their experiences with the larger group.

ADDITIONAL RESOURCES

American Diabetes Association, website: *www.diabetes.org*
American Thyroid Association, website: *www.thyroid.org*
Diabetic Public Health Resource, National Center for Chronic Disease Prevention and Health Promotion, Centers for Disease Control and Prevention, website: *www.cdc.gov/diabetes*
The Endocrine Society, website: *www.endo-society.org*
Juvenile Diabetes Foundation International, website: *www.jdf.org*

CHAPTER 79

Sensory System Disorders

LEARNING OBJECTIVES

1. Describe the parenchymal (functional) structures of the eyes and ears.

2. In the skills lab, demonstrate the technique for obtaining visual acuity using the Snellen chart.

3. Define and differentiate between the following types of testing: refractory error examinations, ophthalmoscope, otoscope, slit lamp, tonometry, ERG, audiometry, caloric test, and ENG. State two nursing considerations for each.

4. In the skills lab, demonstrate a dry wipe and an ear irrigation. Differentiate between the techniques used for adults and children.

5. State at least two reasons for enucleation. Describe the procedure for care of a prosthetic eye.

6. State at least 10 nursing considerations for care of the client with a visual deficit; include pre- and postoperative nursing considerations.

7. State at least 10 nursing considerations for care of the client with a hearing deficit; include pre- and postoperative nursing considerations.

8. Identify at least five NANDA nursing diagnoses for clients with sensory disorders.

9. Define and discuss the following refractory errors: myopia, hyperopia, astigmatism, and presbyopia.

10. Identify the advantages and disadvantages for the following methods of visual correction: eyeglasses, hard contact lenses, soft contact lenses, and extended-wear lenses.

11. Define and discuss the following procedures: radial keratotomy, PKR, and LASIK.

12. Define and differentiate between the following: conjunctivitis, blepharitis, hordeolum, chalazion, trachoma, and keratitis.

13. Differentiate between the following structural disorders: ectropion, entropion, and ptosis.

14. Define and differentiate between chronic open-angle glaucoma, acute closed-angle glaucoma, and secondary glaucoma. Identify at least three nursing considerations for each disorder.

15. Identify the causes and treatments for cataracts. Identify at least three nursing considerations for cataracts.

16. Identify the causes and at least three nursing considerations for each of the following types of eye traumas: contusion and hematoma, foreign bodies, hyphema, chemical burns, corneal abrasions, and detached retina.

17. Define and differentiate between conductive hearing loss, sensorineural hearing loss, central hearing loss, and functional hearing loss.

18. State at least four nursing considerations related to prevention of hearing loss.

19. Discuss the causes and at least two nursing interventions for disorders of the external ear, such as impacted ear wax, furuncles, foreign objects, external otitis, fungal infections, and punctured tympanic membranes.

20. Discuss the causes and at least two nursing interventions for disorders of the middle ear, such as otitis media, serous otitis media, acute purulent otitis media, and chronic otitis media.

21. Prepare a nursing care plan for a client who is to go to surgery for a tympanoplasty and myringotomy with insertion of PE tubes.

22. Define the following and state at least two nursing considerations for each: otosclerosis, mastoiditis, tinnitus, stapedectomy, fenestration, and ototoxic.

23. Identify the causes and at least three nursing considerations for a client with Ménière's disease.

24. Identify at least two nursing considerations for clients with tactile, gustatory, and olfactory disorders.

NEW TERMINOLOGY

blepharitis	olfaction
cataract	ophthalmoscope
cerumen	otitis externa
chalazion	otitis media
conjunctivitis	otosclerosis
diplopia	otoscope
ectropion	ototoxic
entropion	phoroptor
enucleation	proprioception
glaucoma	ptosis
gustation	refraction
hyphema	tactile sense
keratoplasty	tinnitus
Ménière's disease	tonometer
myringotomy	tympanoplasty
nystagmus	

KEY POINTS

- The sensory system is important in enabling people to receive information from the surrounding environment.
- Most eye and ear surgeries are done during day surgery, on an outpatient using the operating microscope. Careful client and family teaching enables clients to resume daily activities.
- Refractive disorders result when light rays focus improperly on the retina.
- Clients with visual impairments may use eyeglasses, contact lenses, and large print materials to enhance their sight.
- Visually impaired individuals can learn to read Braille, listen to books on tape, work with seeing-eye dogs, and use white canes.
- Most eye infections can be treated with the application of warm compresses and topical antibiotic ointments.
- Early recognition and treatment of glaucoma are essential to prevent visual changes and blindness.
- Surgery is the required treatment for cataracts.
- Hearing deficits may occur at any age. They are caused by diseases and congenital and environmental factors.
- Determination of the cause of a hearing deficit is important because it may point to a more serious problem.

- Clients with total hearing loss can learn sign language and lip reading. Clients with partial hearing loss may use hearing aids to enhance remaining hearing.

■ Teaching–Learning Strategies

CLASSROOM

1. Ask the students to define the following terms:

entropion	diplopia
enucleation	cataract
otitis	chalazion
ototoxic	conjunctivitis
blepharitis	tinnitus
stye	bony orbit
glaucoma	refraction
ptosis	hyphema

Write the students' responses on the chalkboard or on an overhead transparency.

2. Briefly review diagnostic tests for vision and hearing impairment. Ask the students to share their own personal experiences with clients or family members with sensory disorders.

3. Show the videotape *Causes of Hearing Loss* (18 minutes; available from Films for the Humanities and Sciences, P.O. Box 2053, Princeton, NJ 08543-2053). After the videotape presentation, open the class for questions and discussion.

4. Briefly review types of vision refractive errors. Ask the students to share with the larger class their personal experiences with vision refractive errors.

5. Assign each pair of students a specific visual, hearing, or other sensory disorder, such as blindness or deafness, and ask the student pairs to formulate a nursing care plan for a client with this disorder. Ask the students to share their care plans with the larger group.

CLINICAL

1. In the clinical laboratory, demonstrate the procedures for dry wipe (ear) and irrigation of the ear. Ask the students to return the demonstration.

2. In the clinical laboratory, divide the students into pairs. Assign one member of each pair to be blind (use a blindfold) or deaf. Ask the students to role

play how they would care for a client with this disorder.

3. On the clinical unit, assign students to clients experiencing a sensory disorder. Assign two or three students to an intensive care setting and work with the nurse caring for clients. Ask the students to interview the nurse about how to decrease sensory overload or deprivation for clients in this setting. Ask the students to share their experiences with the larger group.

4. Ask the students to design a poster to be used to teach preventive techniques for hearing and visual impairments. Ask the students to share their posters with the larger group.

ADDITIONAL RESOURCES

American Foundation for the Blind, 11 Penn Plaza, Suite 300, New York, NY 10001; telephone: 212-202-7600; website: *www.afb.org*

American Speech-Language-Hearing Association, 10801 Rockville Pike, Rockville, MD 20852; telephone: 800-638-8978; website: *www.asha.org*

American Tinnitus Association, P.O. Box 5, Portland, OR 97207; telephone: 800-634-89768; website: *www.ata.org*

Eye Bank Association of America, 1001 Connecticut Avenue, NW, Suite 601, Washington, DC 20036; telephone: 202-775-4999; website: *www.restoresight.org*

Foundation Fighting Blindness, 11435 Cronhill Drive, Owings Mills, MD 21117-2220; telephone: 888-394-3937; website: *www.blindness.org*

Guide Dogs for the Blind, P.O. Box 151200, San Rafael, CA 94915-1200; telephone: 800-295-4050; website: *www.guidedogs.com*

Lions International, 300 West 22nd Street, Oak Brook, IL 60521-8842; telephone: 630-571-5466; website: *www.lions.org*

National Eye Institute, National Institutes of Health, 2020 Vision Place, Bethesda, MD 20892-3655; telephone: 301-496-5248; website: *www.nei.nih.gov*

National Institute on Deafness and Other Communication Disorders, National Institutes of Health, 31 Center Drive, MSC, 2320, Bethesda, MD 20892-2320; telephone: 301-496-7243; website: *www.nidcd.nih.gov*

Prevent Blindness America, 500 East Remington Road, Schaumburg, IL 60173; telephone: 800-331-2020; website: *www.preventblindness.org*

Self Help for Hard of Hearing People, Inc., 7910 Woodmont Avenue, Suite 1200, Bethesda, MD 20814; telephone: 301-657-2248; website: *www.shhh.org*

CHAPTER 80

Cardiovascular Disorders

LEARNING OBJECTIVES

1. Explain the rationales for ordering the following laboratory tests: CPK, CPK-MB, LDH, AST, troponin, and lipid levels.

2. Define and differentiate between an angiocardiogram and an arteriogram. State at least three nursing considerations for these procedures.

3. State the rationale for performing an echocardiogram, an ECG stress test, and an electrophysiology study. Explain the role of the nurse during and after these procedures.

4. State two rationales for obtaining a cardiac catheterization. Identify at least four nursing considerations before and after this procedure.

5. Identify at least six contraindications that would prohibit the use of thrombolytic therapy.

6. Identify the rationale for performing a PTCA.

7. Define and differentiate between closed-heart surgery, open-heart surgery, heart valve replacement, and heart transplantation. Identify at least five postoperative nursing interventions for these procedures.

8. Identify at least five NANDA diagnoses related to the client with a cardiovascular disease or disorder.

9. Define and differentiate between arteriosclerosis and atherosclerosis.

10. Define hypertension and malignant hypertension and discuss at least four complications of hypertensive heart disease.

11. Discuss four common causes of hypotension.

12. Define and differentiate between the following: sinus tachycardia, sinus bradycardia, PVC, heart block, and fibrillation.

13. Discuss the rationale for the use of external and internal defibrillation devices.

14. Identify four possible causes of congestive heart failure.

15. State at least five signs and symptoms of CHF. Relate nursing care to each sign and symptom.

16. Define and differentiate between myocarditis, endocarditis, and pericarditis.

17. Identify four major causes of coronary artery disease.

18. Define and state three signs and symptoms for angina pectoris and myocardial infarction. State four nursing interventions for each condition.

19. Differentiate between the following: thrombophlebitis, deep venous thrombosis, phlebitis, and embolism.

20. Differentiate between intermittent claudication, Buerger's disease, and Raynaud's phenomenon. State three nursing considerations for each disorder.

21. Identify the three main causes of cerebrovascular accidents.

22. State at least four common complications of CVAs.

23. Identify at least six nursing interventions that are important during the various phases of a CVA.

NEW TERMINOLOGY

ablation	fibrillation
aneurysm	heart block
angina pectoris	hemianopsia
angioplasty	hemiplegia
aphasia	hypertrophy
arrhythmia	ischemia
atherectomy	myocarditis
cardiac catheterization	pericarditis
cardioversion	phlebitis
claudication	stenosis
dysrhythmia	stent
echocardiography	thrombolytic
embolus	thrombophlebitis
endocarditis	

KEY POINTS

- Cardiovascular disorders include conditions that interfere with the heart's rhythm, the heart's pumping ability, and those that disrupt the blood flow within the coronary, peripheral, or cerebral arteries.
- Hypertension can lead to such serious problems as myocardial infarction, kidney damage, congestive heart failure, and cerebrovascular accident.
- Some types of heart disease can be cured, whereas others can be controlled by medical or surgical treatment.
- Coronary artery disease develops over many years, so prevention of controllable risk factors should begin early in life.
- Angina or angina pectoris is a temporary loss of oxygen to the heart muscle. If this loss of oxygen supply continues, the result is ischemia (or prolonged deficiency of oxygenated blood), whereas death of heart tissue is called myocardial necrosis.
- Clients who report chest pains should be medicated promptly as ordered by the physician to prevent additional extension of damage to heart muscle caused by anoxia (lack of oxygen).
- Congestive heart failure means the heart is failing, has lost its pumping ability, and is unable to do its work. It is a syndrome (group of symptoms) that affects individuals in different ways and to different degrees.
- Hearing and vision usually are impaired on the person's affected side after a CVA; thus, approach the client from the nonaffected side.

■ Teaching–Learning Strategies

CLASSROOM

1. Ask the students to define the following terms and abbreviations:

hemianopsia	aphasia
thrombophlebitis	angioplasty
CVA	angina pectoris
aneurysm	hemiplegia
Buerger's disease	myocarditis
embolism	congestive heart failure
phlebitis	pericarditis
stroke	claudication
cardiac catheterization	heart block

Write the students' responses on the chalkboard or on an overhead transparency.

2. Review the various tests used to diagnose cardiovascular disorders. Show the videotape(s)

Diagnosing Heart Disease (18 minutes) and *Mending a Heart Without Bypass Surgery* (33 minutes; available from Films for the Humanities and Sciences, P.O. Box 2053, Princeton, NJ 08543-2053). After the videotape presentation(s), open the class for questions and discussion.

3. Invite a nurse who cares for clients with cardiac or cerebrovascular disorders to share with the class about the role of the nurse in caring for these clients. After the presentation, open the class for questions and discussion.

4. Briefly review various cardiovascular disorders and their medical and surgical management. Ask pairs of students to develop a nursing care plan for a client with a specific cardiovascular disorder, such as myocardial infarction, and share their care plans with the larger group.

CLINICAL

1. In the learning laboratory, role play a scenario with students. Ask one student to be the nurse and the other to be a client who has experienced a myocardial infarction. After the role-playing exercise, open the class for questions and discussion.

2. In the clinical setting, assign students to work with a nurse who is caring for clients experiencing a cardiovascular disorder. Ask the students to share their experiences with the larger group.

3. Assign pairs of students to visit a cardiovascular diagnostic center. Ask the students to share their experiences and observations with the larger group.

4. Assign students to a clinical setting that is used for cardiac or stroke rehabilitation. Assign students to work with a staff nurse in the setting. Ask the students to share their experiences with the larger group and demonstrate their nursing care plans.

ADDITIONAL RESOURCES

American Heart Association, website: *www.americanheart.org*
Cardio Info Innovations, website: *www.cardio-info.com*
Heart Center Online for Patients, website: *www.heartcenteronline.com*
National Heart, Lung, Blood Institute, NHLBI Information Center, website: *www.nhlbi.nih.gov*

CHAPTER 81

Blood and Lymph Disorders

LEARNING OBJECTIVES

1. Review the components and functions of the hematologic and lymphatic systems.

2. Explain how different laboratory blood tests can aid in the diagnosis of various problems and disorders.

3. List the various blood components and products used in transfusions.

4. Discuss the importance of blood typing and crossmatching in blood transfusions.

5. Describe symptoms of a transfusion reaction and associated nursing care.

6. Identify diseases in which bone marrow and peripheral stem cell transplantations are used.

7. Describe what is meant by *anemia*; describe its different types and treatments.

8. Describe different types of leukemia and treatments and prognosis for each.

9. Name several platelet and clotting disorders and their signs and symptoms.

10. Differentiate between Hodgkin's disease and non-Hodgkin's lymphoma.

NEW TERMINOLOGY

agranulocytosis	Hodgkin's disease
allogeneic	leukemia
autologous	leukopenia
bone marrow biopsy	oncologist
hematology	sickle cell anemia
hemophilia	thrombocytopenia

KEY POINTS

- Several laboratory blood tests provide indicators of various disorders.

- Blood transfusion is a common treatment for blood disorders. It can cause serious reactions and requires careful nursing observation.
- Bone marrow and peripheral stem cell transplantations are used to treat several life-threatening conditions.
- Anemias deprive a person of energy and oxygen to carry out the activities of daily living.
- White blood cell disorders can affect a person's ability to fight infections.
- Blood disorders affecting clotting factors can cause serious and life-threatening bleeding problems.

■ Teaching–Learning Strategies

CLASSROOM

1. Ask the students to define the following terms and abbreviations:

leukemia	leukopenia
anemia	allogeneic
Hodgkin's disease	bone marrow
thalassemia	thrombocytopenia
pernicious	biopsy
aplastic anemia	DIC
agranulocytosis	lymphoma
hematology	

Write the students' responses on the chalkboard or on an overhead transparency.

2. Briefly review diagnostic tests and medical or surgical treatments for blood and lymph disorders. Assign pairs of students a specific diagnosis, such as leukemia. Ask the students to develop a nursing care plan for clients with these disorders. Ask the students to share their nursing care plans with the larger group.

3. Show the videotape(s) *Administering Blood and Blood Products* (1995; 30 minutes) and *Blood Administration* (available from Insight Media, P.O. Box 621, New York, NY 10024). After the videotape presentation(s), open the class for questions and discussion.

4. Ask a nurse who cares for clients with leukemia to visit the class and present the role of the nurse in caring for these clients. After the presentation, open the class for questions and discussion.

CLINICAL

1. Instruct the students to locate in the clinical setting the policy for administration of blood or blood products. Ask the students to share their findings in clinical conference.

2. Assign students to work in the clinical setting with a nurse who is caring for clients who are experiencing blood or lymph disorders. Ask the students to share their experiences and nursing care plans with the larger group.

3. Ask the students to locate at least one article on the topic of blood or lymph disorders. The library or the Internet can be used. Ask the students to write a one-page summary of the article and share their findings with the larger group.

4. Assign two students to observe a bone marrow or lymph biopsy. If possible, assign students to observe a stem cell transplant. After the procedures, ask the students to share their experiences with the larger group.

ADDITIONAL RESOURCES

American Cancer Society, 1599 Clifton Road NE, Atlanta, GA 30329; telephone: 404-320-3433; website: *www.cancer.org*

American Heart Association National Center, 7372 Greenville Avenue, Dallas, TX 75231; telephone: 800-AHA-USA1; website: *www.americanheart.org*

National Hemophilia Foundation, 110 Green Street, Room 303, New York, NY 10012; telephone: 212-219-8180 or 800-424-2634; website: *www.hemophilia.org*

Sickle Cell Disease Association of America, 200 Corporate Point Suite 495, Culver City, CA 90230-8727; telephone: 800-421-8453; website: *www.sicklecelldisease.org*

CHAPTER 82

Cancer

LEARNING OBJECTIVES

1. Define the terms *carcinoma*, *sarcoma*, *leukemia*, and *lymphoma*.

2. List five factors believed to contribute to cancer.

3. List the seven danger signals of cancer.

4. Identify the four major treatments for cancer.

5. Describe nursing care related to each of the four major types of cancer treatments.

6. Discuss emotional aspects of cancer and appropriate nursing interventions.

7. Explain the specific nutritional needs of the client with cancer.

NEW TERMINOLOGY

adjuvant therapy	malignant
antineoplastic	metastasis
benign	myelosuppression
biopsy	neoplasm
biotherapy	neutropenia
cancer	oncology
carcinogen	palliative
carcinoma	Pap test
chemotherapy	prognosis
cytology	replication
leukemia	sarcoma
lymphoma	

KEY POINTS

- Cancer is an abnormal acceleration of cell growth (uncontrolled, progressive replication).
- Cancer can affect any body system. It can spread to nearby tissues or can metastasize throughout the body.
- The four major types of cancer are carcinoma, sarcoma, leukemia, and lymphoma.
- Many cancers can be cured if they are detected early.

- Cancer is treated by chemicals/medications (chemotherapy), biotherapy (immunotherapy), radiation therapy (external or internal), and surgery.
- The leading cause of cancer death is lung cancer, which often is caused by smoking.
- All persons should learn the seven warning signs of cancer.
- Special nursing care is required by clients undergoing chemotherapy or radiation therapy.

■ Teaching–Learning Strategies

CLASSROOM

1. Ask the students to define the following terms:

alopecia	leukemia
metastasis	Pap test
biotherapy	palliative
chemotherapy	biotherapy
adjuvant therapy	radiation
antineoplastic	lymphoma
biopsy	oncology
benign	neutropenia
malignant	carcinogen
melanoma	sarcoma

Write the students' responses on the chalkboard or on an overhead transparency.

2. Show one or more of the following videotapes during class: *Cancer* (23 minutes), *New Therapies for Cancer* (33 minutes), and *Cancer and Metastasis* (all available from Films for the Humanities and Sciences, P.O. Box 2053, Princeton, NJ 08543-2053). After videotape presentations(s), open the class for questions and discussion.

3. Assign students in pairs to develop a nursing care plan for a client receiving either chemotherapy or radiation. Ask the students to share their care plans with the larger class.

4. Invite a nurse who cares for clients with cancer to visit the class and present the role of the nurse in caring for such clients.

CLINICAL

1. In the clinical setting, assign students to work with a nurse who is caring for clients with the diagnosis of cancer. Ask students to share their nursing care plans and their experiences during clinical conference.

2. Assign students to observe clients receiving radiation therapy or chemotherapy. Ask the students to develop a teaching plan for these clients and share their plans with the larger group.

3. Assign a small number of students to observe in an operating room setting for a client who is having surgical removal of a tumor. Ask students to share their care plans and experiences with the larger group.

4. Assign students to locate one article related to cancer and to write a one- to two-page paper summarizing the article. Ask students to share their papers with the larger group.

5. Assign students to research available (local) community services (e.g., Little Red Door) to assist clients with cancer diagnoses. Ask the students to share their findings with the larger group.

ADDITIONAL RESOURCES

American Cancer Society, 1599 Clifton Road NE, Atlanta, GA 30329; telephone: 404-320-3333; website: *www.cancer.org*

Candlelighters Childhood Cancer Foundation, P.O. Box 498, Kensington, MD 20895; telephone: 800-366-2223; website: *www.candlelighters.org*

Leukemia and Lymphoma Society, 1311 Mamaroneck Avenue, White Plains, NY 10605; telephone: 914-949-5213; website: *www.leukemia.org*

National Alliance of Breast Cancer Associations, 9 East 37th Street, New York, NY 10016; telephone: 212-899-0606; website: *www.nabco.org*

National Cancer Institute, Building 31, Room 10A24, 31 Center Drive, MSC 2580, National Institutes of Health, Bethesda, MD 20892-2580; telephone: 800-4-CANCER; website: *www.nci.nih.gov*

National Coalition for Cancer Survivorship, 1010 Wayne Avenue, Suite 770, Silver Spring, MD 20910-5600; telephone: 301-650-9127 or 877-622-7937; website: *www.cansearch.org*

CHAPTER 83

Allergic, Immune, and Autoimmune Disorders

LEARNING OBJECTIVES

1. Define and differentiate *allergy, antigen, immunogens, antibody,* and *histamine.*

2. Demonstrate the procedure for intradermal skin testing.

3. Discuss at least three components of the medical history and the physical examination that relate to the detection of allergies.

4. State at least five NANDA diagnoses related to the signs and symptoms of allergic disorders.

5. State three possible skin manifestations of the allergic response.

6. State three possible respiratory manifestations of the allergic response.

7. Discuss at least five possible gastrointestinal manifestations of the allergic response.

8. Discuss at least three possible manifestations of the allergic response that relate to drugs.

9. State three methods of treatment for multisystem allergy response.

10. Discuss at least five nursing considerations related to prevention and treatment of anaphylaxis.

11. Differentiate between organ-specific and nonorgan-specific autoimmune diseases.

NEW TERMINOLOGY

allergen	immunity
allergy	immunogen
anaphylaxis	immunosuppression
angioedema	immunotherapy
antibody	induration
antigen	nonorgan specific
autoimmunity	organ specific
eczema	symptomatic
histamine	systemic
hives	urticaria

KEY POINTS

- The immune system leads the "battle" against invading microbes and malignant cells that contact or enter the body.
- The major defenders include T lymphocytes and B cells, which react to antigens by secreting antibodies.
- Antigens are foreign protein substances that enter the body and stimulate the production of antibodies.
- Individuals can be allergic to almost anything.
- Common manifestations of allergic reactions vary; they may range from mild to life threatening (anaphylaxis).
- Treatment of allergies is directed toward removal of the allergen and counteracting the antibody response.
- The body continually seeks a balance between suppressing the immune response that is causing an illness and maintaining enough immunity to fight the invasion of threatening foreign substances.
- Autoimmune disorders occur when the body fails to recognize its own cells as "self" and begins to destroy those cells.

■ Teaching–Learning Strategies

CLASSROOM

1. Ask students to define the following terms:

allergen	histamine
urticaria	eczema
allergy	contact dermatitis
nonorgan specific	antihistamine
antibody	systemic
arthritis	thyrotoxicosis
anaphylaxis	scleroderma
autoimmunity	multiple sclerosis
rejection	bronchospasm
angioedema	

Write the students' responses on the chalkboard or on an overhead transparency.

2. Invite a nurse who works in an allergy clinic to visit the class and discuss the role of the nurse in caring for clients with allergies. After the presentation, open the class for questions and discussion.

3. Ask students to compare and contrast the differences among contact dermatitis, allergic asthma, and allergic rhinitis. Ask the students to identify the steps the nurse should take if a client experiences anaphylaxis.

4. Ask students to research the Internet or a drug textbook for drugs that are used to treat allergies, immune, or autoimmune disorders. Ask the students to share their findings with the larger group.

CLINICAL

1. Assign students to visit a clinic where allergy testing and treatment are performed. After the experience, ask students to share their observations during clinical conference.

2. Assign students to work with a nurse who is caring for a client, in an inpatient setting, with an autoimmune or immune disorder. After the experience, ask students to share their observations during clinical conference.

3. Ask students to research their local community for resources that can be used for clients with these disorders. Ask if there are support groups available for these clients and their families. Ask the students to share their findings with the larger group.

4. Assign students to occupational therapy or physical therapy settings that care for clients with autoimmune disorders, such as rheumatoid arthritis. Ask the students to share their observations with the larger group.

ADDITIONAL RESOURCES

American Academy of Allergy, Asthma and Immunology, website: *www.aaaai.org*

Asthma and Allergy Foundation of America, telephone: 800-7-asthma; E-mail: *info@aafa.org*

Latex Allergy News, website: *www.latexallergyhelp.com.* Other latex allergy resources: *www.latexallergylinks.tripod.com; www.dermadoctor.com*

National Institute of Allergy and Infectious Diseases, website: *www.niaid.nih.gov*

National Jewish Medical and Research Center, website: *www.asthmainkids.com*

CHAPTER 84

HIV and AIDS

LEARNING OBJECTIVES

1. Define a retrovirus, HIV, and AIDS.

2. State at least four routes of transmission for the virus.

3. Discuss the critical nature of the T cells and B cells on the immune system.

4. Describe how HIV targets and invades CD 4 cells.

5. Differentiate between the ELISA and Western blot testing for HIV.

6. State at least eight common signs and symptoms of HIV.

7. Identify at least four signs and symptoms of HIV specific to women.

8. State the three classes of antiretroviral drugs used to treat HIV.

9. Define viral load and differentiate between the technical diagnosis of HIV and AIDS.

10. Describe and discuss at least six opportunistic infections associated with HIV/AIDS.

NEW TERMINOLOGY

acquired immunodeficiency syndrome
AIDS dementia complex
antiretroviral therapy
HIV encephalopathy
human immunodeficiency virus
opportunistic infections
pandemic
Pneumocystis carinii pneumonia
prophylaxis
retrovirus
T cells
viral load

KEY POINTS

- The terms HIV and AIDS are not synonymous. HIV causes AIDS, but the person who has HIV does not automatically have AIDS.
- The Centers for Disease Control and Prevention has updated the definition of AIDS to include diagnosis based on a T-cell count of less than 200 cells/mm^3 blood.
- Follow Standard Precautions in caring for all clients, to protect yourself and minimize the risk of contracting HIV and other infections, such as hepatitis B and C.
- AIDS is ultimately a terminal condition; the emotional, physical, and financial implications can be enormous.

■ Teaching–Learning Strategies

CLASSROOM

1. Ask students to define the following terms and abbreviations:

AIDS	epidemic
HIV	opportunistic
Kaposi's sarcoma	CDC
retrovirus	ELISA
T cells	*Pneumocystis carinii*
B cells	pneumonia
pandemic	

Write the students' responses on the chalkboard or on an overhead transparency.

2. Show the videotape *Good Nutrition for People with HIV/AIDS* (1995; 6 minutes; available from Lippincott Williams & Wilkins, 530 Walnut Street, Philadelphia, PA 19106). After the videotape presentation, open the class for questions and discussion.

3. Invite a nurse or other health care worker who cares for clients with HIV/AIDS to visit the class and present the role of the nurse in caring for these clients. After the presentation, open the class for questions and discussion.

CLINICAL

1. While in the clinical setting, ask the students to review the institution's policy on Standard Precautions. Ask the students to share their findings with the clinical group.

2. Assign each student one medication used to treat the symptoms of HIV/AIDS. Ask students to research the drug, dosage, potential side effects, and nursing implications. Ask the students to share their findings with the larger group.

3. Ask students to research services provided in the local community for clients with HIV/AIDS (and their families). Ask students to share their findings with the larger group.

4. In the clinical laboratory, ask students to practice Standard Precautions with a partner. Use a role-playing scenario in which one of the students is the nurse and the other is the client. After the exercise, open the class for questions and discussion.

ADDITIONAL RESOURCES

Centers for Disease Control and Prevention, website (with links to statistics and other sites, as well as educational materials): *www.cdc.gov*

Hearing-Impaired AIDS Hotline, telephone: 800-243-7889

Information about HIV/AIDS, website: *www.aegis.com*

Kaiser Family Foundation, website (with informational updates and educational materials): *www.kff.org*

National AIDS Information Clearing House, telephone: 800-458-5231

National HIV and AIDS Hotline (CDC), telephone: 800-342-AIDS

Spanish AIDS Hotline, telephone: 800-344-7432

U.S. Public Health Service, telephone: 303-245-6867

CHAPTER 85

Respiratory Disorders

LEARNING OBJECTIVES

1. State the rationale for the use of each of the following laboratory tests: sputum, lavage, throat culture, and ABG.

2. State the rationale for the use of each of the following: CXR, CT, MRI, lung scan, lung perfusion scan, pulmonary angiography, and PFT.

3. Identify at least four reasons for skin testing.

4. Demonstrate the positions of postural drainage.

5. Differentiate between the following: thoracentesis, paracentesis, and thoracotomy.

6. Identify at least four nursing considerations related to closed water seal drainage.

7. Identify at least five alterations in normal respiratory status.

8. Identify the nursing concerns of each type of hypoxia.

9. Identify at least 10 interventions that can assist the client who is in respiratory distress.

10. Define and differentiate between the following infectious respiratory disorders: acute rhinitis, streptococcal throat infection, influenza, laryngitis, bronchitis, lung abscesses, pneumonia, pleurisy, histoplasmosis, tuberculosis, and empyema.

11. Define and differentiate between the following chronic obstructive pulmonary diseases: asthma, bronchiectasis, bronchitis, and emphysema.

12. Identify three nursing considerations for a client with ARDS.

13. State three common sources of trauma to the lungs and identify three nursing considerations for each.

14. Differentiate between benign and malignant lung disorders.

15. Identify three common inflammatory disorders of the nose.

16. Identify four structural disorders of the nose.

17. Identify three considerations of nursing care for epistaxis.

NEW TERMINOLOGY

anergic	pleurisy
asphyxiation	pneumonectomy
asthma	pneumonia
atelectasis	pneumothorax
bronchiectasis	postural drainage
bronchitis	pulmonary emphysema
bronchoscopy	rhinitis
empyema	rhinoplasty
epistaxis	sinusitis
hemothorax	strangulation
hyperventilation	suffocation
incentive spirometer	thoracentesis
laryngectomy	tracheostomy
lobectomy	tuberculosis
paracentesis	

KEY POINTS

- The respiratory and cardiovascular systems are vital to the entire body's functioning because they provide and transport oxygen to cells and wastes away from cells.
- Nursing assessment of a client with a respiratory disorder is critical in determining the severity of respiratory distress, the immediacy of the situation, and necessary care.
- Disorders of the respiratory system may be caused by infections (bacteria, virus, fungi), irritants (smoking, allergens, environmental chemicals), masses (cancerous tumors), or trauma.
- Respiratory disorders may be characterized by multiple clinical manifestations such as cough, changes in respiratory pattern, and abnormal breath sounds.

- When hypoxia (lack of oxygen) occurs, subsequent changes in the neurologic and cardiovascular systems may develop.
- Key elements in the treatment of respiratory disorders include medications specific to the disease; oxygen administration; postural drainage; positioning; turning, coughing, and deep breathing; and breathing exercises.
- The goals of nursing management for persons with respiratory disorders are a patent (open) airway, effective breathing pattern, and improved gas exchange.

■ Teaching–Learning Strategies

CLASSROOM

1. Ask students to define the following terms and abbreviations:

hemothorax	postural drainage
laryngectomy	rhinoplasty
bronchoscopy	sleep apnea syndrome
empyema	pleurisy
epistaxis	pneumonia
trauma	sinusitis
anergic	tuberculosis
hyperventilation	strangulation
rhinitis	COPD
asphyxiation	allergy
asthma	pulmonary
bronchitis	emphysema
paracentesis	

Write the students' responses on the chalkboard or on an overhead transparency.

2. Before class, on 3 × 5 index cards, write a respiratory disorder (e.g., pneumonia) on each card. During class, ask the students to join in pairs. Give each pair an index card with a disorder and ask the students to develop a nursing care plan for a client with this disorder. Ask the students to share their findings with the larger group.

3. Show the videotape *Pathophysiology of Chronic Obstructive Pulmonary Disease* (1997; available from Lippincott Williams & Wilkins, 530 Walnut Street, Philadelphia, PA 19106). After the videotape presentation, open the class for questions and discussion.

4. Ask a volunteer or a nurse who works for the American Lung Association to visit the class and discuss prevention strategies for respiratory disorders. After the presentation, open the class for questions and discussion.

CLINICAL

1. Assign students to provide care, in the clinical setting, for a client with a respiratory disorder. Ask the students to share their nursing care plans for the client during clinical conference.

2. Ask the students to use the Internet or the library to locate one article that relates to respiratory disorders. Ask the students to write a one- to two-page summary of the article.

3. Assign each student a specific drug to research. Ask the students to present their findings during clinical conference.

4. Ask students to research their local community for support services available to clients with respiratory disorders. Ask the students to share their findings during clinical conference.

5. Ask students to divide into pairs and develop a poster on the topic of prevention of respiratory disorders for various age groups. Ask students to share their posters with the larger group. Donate the posters to an appropriate facility.

ADDITIONAL RESOURCES

American Lung Association, website: *www.lungusa.org*
Asthma and Allergy Foundation of America, website: *www.aafa.org*
Centers for Disease Control and Prevention, website: *www.cdc.gov/health/diseases*
Cystic Fibrosis Foundation, 6931 Arlington Road, Bethesda, MD 20814; telephone: 800-FIGHT-CF
National Heart, Lung, and Blood Institute, website: *www.nhlbi.nih.gov*
National Jewish Center for Immunology and Respiratory Medicine, website: *www.nationaljewish.org*
National Tuberculosis Center, website: *www.umdnj.edu/ntbcweb*

CHAPTER 86

Oxygen Therapy and Respiratory Care

LEARNING OBJECTIVES

1. State the three major goals of oxygen therapy.

2. Discuss at least four key safety factors and hazards in oxygen administration.

3. Describe the use of the pulse oximeter.

4. Identify at least five sources of oxygen and describe how they differ.

5. List at least eight key points in nursing assessment of the client who is receiving oxygen.

6. Describe and differentiate the types of oxygen delivery systems, including simple mask, partial-rebreathing mask, nonrebreathing mask, Venturi mask, IPPB, aerosol mist treatment, and a manual breathing bag.

7. State at least three key safety factors /or nursing considerations with the use of each of the oxygen delivery systems.

8. Demonstrate how to set up basic oxygen equipment.

9. Discuss at least five nursing considerations for the client receiving oxygen, using mechanical ventilation, or with a tracheostomy.

NEW TERMINOLOGY

hyperbaric	respirator
manual breathing bag (Ambu bag)	simple mask
	tracheostomy
nasal cannula	ventilator
nonrebreathing mask	Venturi mask
pulse oximeter	

KEY POINTS

- Oxygen is essential to life. Without oxygen, a person will die in a matter of minutes.

- Therapeutic oxygen is like a medication. It requires a physician's prescription and has associated safety considerations that you must understand and follow.
- Oxygen supports combustion; you must take great care when using oxygen because a fire can start and be explosive.
- Oxygen administration can assist a person to breathe or can totally support life.
- Oxygen is administered to support breathing in several ways: nasal cannula, simple mask, partial-rebreathing mask, nonrebreathing mask, Venturi mask, intermittent positive pressure breathing, and aerosol mist.
- Manual breathing bags, ventilators, and tracheostomy tubes are methods of assisting the person to breathe who cannot do so on his or her own.
- The nurse works with the respiratory care professionals in oxygen administration.

■ Teaching–Learning Strategies

CLASSROOM

1. Ask students to define the following terms:

pulse oximeter	flow meter
Venturi mask	strollers
respirator	nasal cannula
concentration	hyperbaric chamber
oxygen cylinder	nonrebreathing mask
partial-rebreathing mask	aerosol mist humidifier
	ventilator
tracheostomy	Ambu bag
regulator	obturator

Write the students' responses on the chalkboard or on an overhead transparency.

2. Bring various types of oxygen equipment to class for demonstration. Ask the students to share their personal experiences with clients receiving oxygen.

3. Show the videotape(s) *Respiratory Therapy in the Home* (1993; 25 minutes) and *Tracheostomy Care* (1992; 28 minutes; both available from Lippincott Williams & Wilkins, 530 Walnut Street, Philadelphia, PA 19106). After the videotape presentation(s), open the class for questions and discussion.

4. Invite a nurse who provides home care to clients receiving oxygen to visit the class and discuss the experiences of providing oxygen therapy in the home setting. After the presentation, open the class for questions and discussion.

CLINICAL

1. In the learning laboratory, demonstrate the equipment used for provision of oxygen and

suctioning a tracheostomy. Ask the students to practice the skills on a model.

2. Ask the students to use the Internet or the library to locate one article related to oxygen therapies. Ask the students to write a one- to two-page summary of the article and share their findings with the larger group.

3. In the clinical setting, assign students to work with a nurse who is caring for a client receiving oxygen or who has a tracheostomy. Ask students to share their nursing care plans during clinical conference.

4. Assign small groups of students to an intensive care setting where the clients are receiving oxygen. Ask students to share their observations with the larger group.

CHAPTER 87

Digestive Disorders

LEARNING OBJECTIVES

1. Review the anatomy and physiology of the gastrointestinal system.

2. Identify common x-ray and direct visualization examinations used to diagnose GI disorders and describe the nursing considerations for each.

3. Explain the purpose and process of gastric suction and gavage.

4. Describe nursing care of the client with a nasogastric tube.

5. Describe common structural, inflammatory, infectious, traumatic, and neoplastic disorders of the mouth and indicate treatment and nursing considerations for each.

6. Describe common structural, inflammatory, and neoplastic disorders of the esophagus and indicate nursing considerations for each.

7. Discuss the causes, signs and symptoms, treatment, nursing considerations, and complications of stomach ulcers.

8. Describe the pre- and postoperative nursing care when the client has gastric surgery and identify potential postoperative complications.

9. Discuss the signs, symptoms, and treatment of stomach cancer.

10. Describe common structural, functional, inflammatory, and neoplastic disorders of the small and large intestine and indicate treatment and nursing considerations for each.

11. Discuss the nursing care and teaching implications when the client has an ostomy.

12. Identify common chronic and inflammatory disorders of the liver and indicate treatment and nursing considerations for each.

13. Describe common inflammatory and neoplastic disorders of the gallbladder and pancreas.

14. Describe causes, complications, treatment, and nursing considerations for problems of overnutrition and undernutrition.

NEW TERMINOLOGY

achalasia	hemorrhoids
adhesions	hepatitis
anastomosis	hernia
appendicitis	ileostomy
ascites	inflammatory bowel disease
bruxism	intussusception
cachexia	leukoplakia buccalis
caries	melena
cholelithiasis	paracentesis
cirrhosis	paralytic ileus
colonoscopy	peritonitis
colostomy	pilonidal cyst
diverticulitis	polypectomy
dumping syndrome	pyorrhea
dyspepsia	steatorrhea
esophagoscopy	stoma
evisceration	tenesmus
fistula	ulcer
gastrectomy	varices
gastritis	volvulus
gastroscopy	

KEY POINTS

- The GI tract is responsible for the digestion of food, absorption of nutrients, and elimination of metabolic waste material.
- Diagnostic tests for disorders of the GI tract include serum liver enzymes, blood urea nitrogen, creatinine, and blood coagulation studies. Invasive testing of the GI tract includes endoscopies, EGD, and ERCP.
- Nursing care of the client with a digestive disorder includes management of nasogastric tubes (e.g., lavage, suction, irrigation), stoma care (e.g., colostomies and ileostomies), and the ability to obtain data concerning nutritional history and disorders.

- Ulcers can be found in both the stomach and duodenum. Surgical intervention may be necessary to prevent or treat hemorrhage; however, medications also are effective in ulcer management.
- Irritable bowel syndrome is annoying and usually treated symptomatically. Inflammatory bowel diseases such as ulcerative colitis and Crohn's disease are long-term, progressive, and often life-threatening.
- The liver is subject to several forms of debilitating illness. Toxins, drugs, and many viruses can result in acute forms of hepatitis. Alcohol is related to cirrhosis and esophageal varices.
- Diseases of the accessory organs of the GI tract include cholecystitis, cholelithiasis, pancreatitis, and appendicitis.
- Cancer of many areas of the GI tract often is not found until metastasis has occurred. Common signs of GI cancer include alterations in eating habits and bowel elimination, weight loss, and rectal bleeding.

■ Teaching–Learning Strategies

CLASSROOM

1. Ask students to define the following terms:

volvulus	cachexia
ulcer	ascites
peptic	cirrhosis
endoscopy	dysphagia
achalasia	colostomy
adhesions	lavage
melena	hernia
fistula	ileostomy
nasogastric	paracentesis
anastomosis	steatorrhea

Write the students' responses on the chalkboard or on an overhead transparency.

2. Before class, on 3 × 5 index cards, write a specific digestive disorder (e.g., peptic ulcer) on each card. During the class, assign students in pairs to develop a nursing care plan for a client with this disorder. Ask the students to share their care plans with the larger group.

3. Invite a nurse who cares for clients with ostomies to visit the class and explain the role of the nurse in caring for these clients. After the presentation, open the class for questions and discussion.

4. Show the videotape *Ostomy Care* (1993; 24 minutes; available from Insight Media, P.O. Box 621, New York, NY 10024). After the videotape presentation, open the class for questions and discussion.

5. Ask students to share their experiences in working with clients who have a digestive disorder.

CLINICAL

1. Assign small groups of students to assist in the endoscopy department or to observe procedures in the operating room for clients with digestive disorders. Ask the students to share their observations with the larger group.

2. Ask students to locate an article using the Internet or the library that relates to digestive disorders. Ask the students to write a one- to two-page paper summarizing the article. Ask the students to share their findings with the larger group.

3. In the clinical setting, assign students to work with a nurse who is caring for clients with digestive disorders. Ask the students to share their nursing care plans with the larger group.

4. In the learning laboratory, have pairs of students role-play. One student in each pair can be the client with a specific digestive disorder, such as hepatitis, while the other is the nurse. After the role-playing exercise, open the class for questions and discussion.

ADDITIONAL RESOURCES

American Gastroenterology Association, 7910 Woodmont Avenue, Seventh floor, Bethesda, MD 20814; telephone: 301-654-2055; website: *www.gastro.org*
American Liver Foundation, 75 Maiden Lane, Suite 603, New York, NY 10038; telephone: 800-465-4837; website: *www.liverfoundation.org*
Colitis and Crohn's Foundation, 386 Park Avenue South, New York, NY 10016-8804; website: *www.ccfa.org*
National Eating Disorders Association, 603 Stewart St., Suite 803, Seattle, WA 98101; telephone: (206) 382-3587; website: *www.nationaleatingdisorders.org*
National Institutes of Diabetes, Digestive and Kidney Disease, National Institutes of Health, Building 31, Room 9A04, Center Drive, MSC 2560, Bethesda, MD 20892-2560; website: *www.niddk.nih.gov*
United Ostomy Association, Inc., 19772 MacArthur Boulevard, Suite 600, Irvine, CA 92612-2405; telephone: 800-826-0826; website: *www.uoa.org*

CHAPTER 88

Urinary Disorders

LEARNING OBJECTIVES

1. List important assessment factors for the urinary system.

2. Describe major urine, blood, imaging and contrast studies, endoscopy, and other diagnostic tests used to evaluate the function of the urinary system.

3. Identify categories of incontinence and treatment goals for each type.

4. Discuss the pathological and treatment differences between cystitis, pyelonephritis, and glomerulonephritis.

5. Describe the nursing considerations when the client has an inflammatory or infectious problem of the bladder and kidneys.

6. Explain the effect of obstructive disorders on urinary and renal function.

7. Describe medical and surgical treatments for stones and nursing considerations.

8. Describe the types of malignancy that occur in the bladder and kidney.

9. Discuss medical and surgical treatments for urinary or renal malignancy.

10. Describe the various types of urinary diversion procedures and describe nursing considerations.

11. Differentiate between acute and chronic renal failure.

12. List the advantages and disadvantages of peritoneal dialysis, hemodialysis, and kidney transplantation.

13. Discuss the nursing considerations when the client is receiving dialysis.

NEW TERMINOLOGY

accommodation	Kegel exercises
anasarca	kidney
anuria	leak point pressure
artificial sphincter	levators
bacteriuria	lithiasis
benign prostatic hypertrophy	lithotripsy
	lower tract
biofeedback	meatus
bladder	medulla
bolus	micturition
calculi	nephrectomy
calices	nephrolithiasis
casts	nephrologist
colic	nephroma
compliance	nephrons
cortex	neurogenic
Crede maneuver	oliguria
crystalluria	overflow/paradoxical
cylindruria	incontinence
cystitis	peristalsis
cystogram	pessary
cystometrogram	prolapse
cystoscopy	pubococcygeal
detrusor	pyelonephritis
dialysis	pyramids
diuresis	pyuria
dome	reflex incontinence
dysuria	reflux
electrical stimulation	renal failure
extracorporeal	renal pelvis
extrophy	residual urine volume
fistula	retention
glomeruli	sensitivity test
glomerulonephritis	shock wave
hematuria	shunt
hemodialysis	sphincters
hemofiltration	stasis
hydrodistention	stent
hydronephrosis	stress incontinence
hypotonic	stricture
iatrogenic incontinence	suprapubic
ileal diversion	symphysis pubis
incontinence	total incontinence
interstitial cystitis	transient incontinence

upper tract
ureter
ureterolithotomy
urethra
urethral pressure profile
urge incontinence

urine
urodynamics/urodynamic
   testing
uroflowmetry
urologist
voiding study

KEY POINTS

- The kidneys are sensitive to disruption of blood flow.
- All body systems affect urinary function. In turn, disorders of the kidneys affect all body systems.
- Most incontinence is treatable.
- Nursing care of the client with a urinary disorder focuses on maintaining and preserving renal function, decreasing discomfort, preventing infection, promoting skin integrity, maintaining fluid balance, and restoring/maintaining the client's self-esteem.
- Early symptoms of renal disease are subtle. The nurse's ability to detect small changes in the client is crucial to early treatment.

▪ Teaching–Learning Strategies

CLASSROOM

1. Ask students to define the following terms:

nephrologist
ileal conduit
pouch
anuria
calculi
hemodialysis
pyuria
cystogram
dialysis
lithotripsy

crystalluria
glomerulonephritis
cystitis
lithiasis
micturition
renal failure
urologist
nephrolithiasis
residual urine volume

Write the students' responses on the chalkboard or on an overhead transparency.

2. Show the videotape *Kidney Disease* (26 minutes; available from Films for the Humanities and Sciences, P.O. Box 2053, Princeton, NJ 08543-2052). After the videotape presentation, open the class for questions and discussion.

3. Invite a nurse who cares for clients receiving hemodialysis to visit the class and present the role of the nurse in caring for these clients. After the presentation, open the class for questions and discussion.

4. Assign each pair of students a specific urinary disorder, such as chronic renal failure. Ask each pair of students to develop a nursing care plan for a client with this disorder. Ask the students to share their nursing care plans with the larger group.

CLINICAL

1. In the learning laboratory, review urinary catheterization if needed. Demonstrate the various pieces of equipment for treating renal disorders (e.g., ileal conduit). After the demonstration, ask the students to demonstrate the skills.

2. Assign small groups of students to a diagnostic setting that is used for clients with urinary disorders. After the observational experience, ask the students to share their observations with the larger group.

3. Assign students to work with a nurse who is caring for clients with urinary disorders. After the experiences, ask the students to share their nursing care plans with the larger group.

4. Instruct the students to use the library or Internet to locate an article on the topic of urinary disorders. Ask the students to write a one- to two-page summary of the article and share their summaries with the larger group.

ADDITIONAL RESOURCES

Agency for Healthcare Research and Quality, P.O. Box 8547, Silver Spring, MD 20907; telephone: 800-358-9295; website: *www.ahrq.gov*

American Cancer Society, 1599 Clifton Road NE, Atlanta, GA 30329-4251; telephone: 800-227-2345; website: *www.cancer.org*

American Foundation for Urologic Disease/Bladder Health Council, 1128 North Charles Street, Baltimore, MD 21201; telephone: 800-242-2383; website: *www.afud.org*

Interstitial Cystitis Association of America, 51 Monroe Street, Rockville, MD 20850; telephone: 800-435-7422; website: *www.ichelp.org*

National Association for Continence, P.O. Box 8310, Spartanburg, SC 29305-8310; telephone: 800-BLADDER (800-252-3337); website: *www.nafc.org*

The National Enuresis Society, 7777 Forest Lane, Suite C-737, Dallas, TX 75230-2518; website: *www.peds.umn.edu/centers/nes*

National Kidney Foundation, 30 East 33rd Street, Suite 1100, New York, NY 10016; telephone: 800-622-9010; website: *www.kidney.org*

National Kidney and Urologic Diseases Information Clearinghouse, 3 Information Way, Bethesda, MD 20892-3580; telephone: 800-891-5390; website: *www.niddk.nih.gov*

National Multiple Sclerosis Society, 733 3rd Avenue, New York, NY 10017; telephone: 800-344-4867; website: *www.nationalmssociety.org*

Spina Bifida Association of America, 4590 MacArthur Boulevard NW, Suite 250, Washington, DC 20007-4226; telephone: 800-621-3141; website: *www.sbaa.org*

United Ostomy Association, 19772 MacArthur Boulevard, Suite 200, Irvine, CA 92612-2405; telephone: 800-826-0826; website: *www.uoa.org*

CHAPTER 89

Male Reproductive Disorders

LEARNING OBJECTIVES

1. Differentiate between the following laboratory tests: testosterone level, PSA level, and a free PSA level.

2. Describe the circumstances that would be necessary for the physician to order an NPT test, a duplex doppler ultrasonography, and a prostatic biopsy.

3. List four nursing diagnoses appropriate for men with reproductive disorders.

4. Differentiate between the medical and surgical treatments for erectile disorders.

5. Define and discuss at least five causes of erectile dysfunction.

6. Define and discuss at least four causes of priapism.

7. Compare and contrast the signs and symptoms of the following: Peyronie's disease, hypospadias, epispadias, cryptorchidism, phimosis, torsion of the spermatic cord, varicocele, and hydrocele.

8. Compare and contrast the signs and symptoms of epididymitis, orchitis, prostatitis (acute and chronic), and nonbacterial prostatitis.

9. Define and differentiate between the signs and symptoms of BPH and cancer of the prostate.

10. In the skills lab, demonstrate a three-way bladder irrigation.

11. Differentiate between the five common surgical approaches to prostatectomy.

12. Discuss at least four postoperative nursing considerations for care of a client with TURP.

13. Discuss the etiologies, signs, and symptoms of prostate cancer as compared with testicular cancer and penile cancer.

14. Prepare a teaching plan for TSE.

NEW TERMINOLOGY

cryptorchidism	orchitis
epididymitis	phimosis
epispadias	plication
hesitancy	priapism
hydrocele	prostatectomy
hyperplasia	prostate specific antigen
hypospadias	prostatitis
impotence	seminoma
nonseminoma	testicular self-examination
orchiopexy	varicocele

KEY POINTS

- Conditions that affect male reproductive function potentially affect body image and self-esteem.
- Erectile dysfunction generally is organic in nature.
- Maintenance of continuous bladder irrigation requires vigilant nursing management.
- Torsion of the spermatic cord is an emergency; if unrelieved, it may cause necrosis of the affected testicle.
- Recurrent or chronic infection of the genitourinary tract may affect fertility.
- There are four types of prostatitis, each with different management strategies.
- Most testicular cancers occur between the ages of 18 and 34 years. All males should perform testicular self-examination from early adolescence onward.
- Inform clients contemplating surgical treatment of benign prostatic hyperplasia that they may experience some incontinence or impotence after surgery.
- All men older than 50 years should have a yearly rectal digital examination and PSA; those with increased risk of prostate cancer should start screening at 45.

■ Teaching–Learning Strategies

CLASSROOM

1. Ask the students to define the following terms
   and abbreviations:

impotence	epididymitis
cryptorchidism	orchiectomy
nonseminoma	orchitis
varicocele	prostatectomy
epispadias	hesitance
hypospadias	spermatic cord
hydrocele	hernia
plication	BPH

   Write the students' responses on the chalkboard
   or on an overhead transparency.

2. Assign each pair of students a specific male
   reproductive disorder. Ask each pair of students
   to develop a nursing care plan for a client with
   the disorder. Ask the students to share their
   nursing care plans with the larger group.

3. Invite a nurse who cares for male clients with
   reproductive disorders to visit the class and
   present the role of the nurse in caring for these
   clients. After the presentation, open the class for
   questions and discussion.

4. Review the procedure for testicular self-
   examination. Ask the students to identify clients
   who need teaching regarding testicular self-
   examination and their rationale.

5. Assign students to use the library or Internet to
   locate an article on the topic of male reproductive
   disorders. Ask the students to write a one- to
   two-page summary of the article and share their
   summaries with the larger group.

CLINICAL

1. In the learning laboratory, demonstrate the
   procedure and equipment for transurethral
   resection of the prostate. Ask students to return
   the demonstration.

2. In the clinical setting, assign small groups of
   students to a diagnostic testing center for clients
   with possible male reproductive disorders. Assign
   small groups of students to an operating room
   setting where they are able to observe a
   prostatectomy being performed. After the
   experiences, ask the students to share their
   observations with the larger group.

3. Assign students to work with a nurse who is
   caring for clients with male reproductive disorders.
   After the experiences, ask students to share their
   nursing care plans with the larger group.{NL}

ADDITIONAL RESOURCES

American Cancer Society, website: *www.cancer.org*
American Foundation for Urological Disease, Inc. (AFUD),
    website: *www.afud.org*
American Urologic Association, website: *www.auanet.org*
National Cancer Institute, website: *www.nci.nih.gov*

CHAPTER 90

Female Reproductive Disorders

LEARNING OBJECTIVES

1. Describe the rationale, procedure, and nursing implications for the following diagnostic tests: pelvic examination, Pap test, breast examination, mammography, breast ultrasound, and ultrasonography.

2. Define and differentiate between the following: laparoscopy, culdoscopy, colposcopy, cervical biopsy, and conization.

3. Describe at least five nursing implications for a client who needs a D&C.

4. Distinguish between the procedures and state the rationale for performing a hysterectomy and pelvic exenteration and between a mammoplasty and mastectomy.

5. List at least eight factors involved in the nursing assessment of a breast or reproductive disorder.

6. Identify at least five common nursing diagnoses for a woman with a breast or reproductive disorder.

7. Relate at least eight teaching components related to each of the following concepts: feminine hygiene and breast self-exam.

8. In the skills lab, demonstrate the following procedures: providing perineal care, providing sitz baths, inserting a vaginal suppository, and performing a douche (vaginal irrigation).

9. Define and differentiate between the following menstrual disorders: amenorrhea, menorrhagia, metrorrhagia, dysmenorrhea, and extreme irregularity.

10. Describe the cause and symptoms of PMS and TSS, including at least three teaching components for nursing care.

11. Identify at least four common client concerns related to menopause and HRT.

12. Define and differentiate between the following structural disorders: vaginal fistula, cystocele, rectocele, prolapsed uterus, and abnormal flexion of the uterus.

13. Define and differentiate the following disorders: vaginitis, trichomonas vaginalis, candidiasis, bacterial vaginosis, atrophic vaginitis, cervicitis, endometriosis, PID, vulvodynia, and STDs.

14. Define and differentiate ovarian cancer, uterine cancer, and cervical cancer.

15. Identify the pre- and postoperative nursing care of a client undergoing an abdominal hysterectomy and a vaginal hysterectomy.

16. Identify the steps of breast self-examination.

17. Explain the pre- and postoperative nursing care of a client undergoing breast biopsy, mastectomy, or reconstructive breast surgery.

NEW TERMINOLOGY

amenorrhea	mammoplasty
cervicitis	mastalgia
conization	mastectomy
culdoscopy	menarche
cystocele	menorrhagia
dilation and curettage	metrorrhagia
dysmenorrhea	Pap test
dyspareunia	prolapse
endometriosis	puberty
gynecology	rectocele
hysterectomy	sentinel lymph node
laparoscopy	toxic shock syndrome
leukorrhea	vaginitis
mammography	vulvitis

KEY POINTS

- A sexual history is important in defining areas of concern.
- Observation of one's own menstrual cycle patterns and breast self-examination are helpful in the early diagnosis of female reproductive disorders.
- Diagnostic studies are necessary (although sometimes uncomfortable) processes. Nurses are

invaluable in preparing the client and relieving her concerns.

- Nursing skills performed to assist the female client include perineal care, vaginal irrigation, and insertion of vaginal suppositories.
- Nurses can assist women to prevent reproductive problems through clear and understandable client teaching.
- Explanation and follow-up with a client who must undergo surgical treatment is important. The client may not have heard or understood all that was explained to her.
- High cure rates exist in certain cancers if discovered early (especially breast and cervical cancer).

▪ Teaching–Learning Strategies

CLASSROOM

1. Ask the students to define the following terms and abbreviations:

vulvitis	mammography
amenorrhea	mastalgia
dysmenorrhea	metrorrhagia
menorrhagia	cysts
cervicitis	gynecology
endometriosis	hysterectomy
culdoscopy	rectocele
pelvic inflammatory disease	vaginitis
	STDs
cystocele	Dilatation and curettage
mammoplasty	

Write the students' responses on the chalkboard or on an overhead transparency.

2. Before class, assign each student to research a specific medication (e.g., metronidazole [Flagyl]) related to female reproductive disorders. Ask students to share their findings about the medication with the larger class.

3. Assign students in pairs to a specific female reproductive disorder (e.g., vaginitis). Ask each pair of students to develop a nursing care plan for a client with this disorder. Ask the students to share their findings with the larger group.

4. Show the videotape(s) *Pathophysiology of Breast Cancer* (1997; 20 minutes) and *Care of the Client with Breast Cancer* (1997; 20 minutes; both available from Lippincott Williams & Wilkins,

530 Walnut Street, Philadelphia, PA 19106). After the videotape presentation(s), open the class for questions and discussion.

CLINICAL

1. Assign students to a gynecology clinic. Ask the students to work with a nurse who is caring for the clients in the clinic. After the experiences, ask the students to share their observations with the larger group.

2. Assign small groups of students to a women's health or diagnostic center that performs diagnostic testing. After the experience, ask students to share their observations with the larger group.

3. In an inpatient setting, assign students to work with a nurse caring for a client undergoing treatment for a female reproductive disorder (e.g., a client with breast cancer who is having a mastectomy). After the experiences, ask students to share their nursing care plans during clinical conference.

4. Ask students in pairs to design a poster related to the topic of breast health and self-examination. Ask the students to share their posters with the larger group. Donate the students' posters to an appropriate clinical site.

5. Ask the students to locate one article related to female reproductive disorders. Ask the students to write a one- to two-page summary of the article and share their summaries with the larger group.

SUGGESTED RESOURCES: VIDEOTAPES

Acute care of burns. (1995). [25 minutes]. (Available from Insight Media, P.O. Box 621, New York, NY 10024)

AIDS: The heart of the matter. (1996). [31 minutes]. (Available from Aquarius Health Care Videos, P.O. Box 1159, Sherborn, MA 01770)

Assessing fluids and electrolytes. (1989). [30 minutes]. (Available from Insight Media, P.O. Box 621, New York, NY 10024)

Assisting with casts and traction. (1992). [73 minutes]. (Available from Insight Media, P.O. Box 621, New York, NY 10024)

Assisting with crutches and walkers. (1992). [37 minutes]. (Available from Insight Media, P.O. Box 621, New York, NY 10024)

Both ends burning. [14 minutes]. (Available from Fanlight Productions, 47 Halifax Street, Boston, MA 02130; 800-937-4113)

Breast cancer: Coping with your diagnosis. [37 minutes]. (Available from Films for the Humanities and Sciences, P.O. Box 2053, Princeton, NJ 08543-2053)

Breast cancer: Recovering from surgery. [30 minutes]. (Available from Films for the Humanities and Sciences, P.O. Box 2053, Princeton, NJ 08543-2053)

Breast cancer: Understanding adjuvant therapy. [30 minutes]. (Available from Films for the Humanities and Sciences, P.O. Box 2053, Princeton, NJ 08543-2053)

Breast cancer: Your ongoing recovery. [30 minutes]. (Available from Films for the Humanities and Sciences, P.O. Box 2053, Princeton, NJ 08543-2053)

Breast health for women over 60. (1995). [14 minutes]. (Available from Aquarius Health Care Videos, P.O. Box 1159, Sherborn, MA 01770)

Care of the patient with pain. (Available from Lippincott Williams & Wilkins, 530 Walnut Street, Philadelphia, PA 19106)

Cataract series. (1989). [3 videos; 19 minutes]. (Available from Lippincott Williams & Wilkins, 530 Walnut Street, Philadelphia, PA 19106)

Catheterization and urinary care. (1993). [24 minutes]. (Available from Insight Media, P.O. Box 621, New York, NY 10024)

IV therapy for pediatric patients. (1995). [18 minutes]. (Available from Lippincott Williams & Wilkins, 530 Walnut Street, Philadelphia, PA 19106)

Living with heart failure. [20 minutes]. (Available from Films for the Humanities and Sciences, P.O. Box 2053, Princeton, NJ 08543-2053)

Pathophysiology of cerebral vascular accident. (1997). (Available from Lippincott Williams & Wilkins, 530 Walnut Street, Philadelphia, PA 19106)

Pathophysiology of heart failure. (1997). (Available from Lippincott Williams & Wilkins, 530 Walnut Street, Philadelphia, PA 19106)

Pediatric AIDS. [21 minutes]. (Available from Films for the Humanities and Sciences, P.O. Box 2053, Princeton, NJ 08543-2053)

Pneumonia: All you need to know. [20 minutes]. (Available from Films for the Humanities and Sciences, P.O. Box 2053, Princeton, NJ 08543-2053)

Preventing a heart attack. [19 minutes]. (Available from Films for the Humanities and Sciences, P.O. Box 2053, Princeton, NJ 08543-2053)

Reservoirs of strength: Burn rehabilitation. (1990). [57 minutes]. (Available from Insight Media, P.O. Box 621, New York, NY 10024)

Respiratory suctioning. (1993). [20 minutes]. (Available from Lippincott Williams & Wilkins, 530 Walnut Street, Philadelphia, PA 19106)

Three days out (breast cancer). (1997). [54 minutes]. (Available from Aquarius Health Care Videos, P.O. Box 1159, Sherborn, MA 01770)

Total knee replacement: Patient education. (1989). [23 minutes]. (Available from Lippincott Williams & Wilkins, 530 Walnut Street, Philadelphia, PA 19106)

Traction: Checks and balances. (1986). [28 minutes]. (Available from Lippincott Williams & Wilkins, 530 Walnut Street, Philadelphia, PA 19106)

ADDITIONAL RESOURCES

American Cancer Society, website: *www.cancer.org*
National Cancer Institute, website: www.*nci.nih.gov*

CHAPTER 91

Gerontology: The Aging Adult

LEARNING OBJECTIVES

1. List at least five care settings for older adults, stating advantages and disadvantages of each.

2. Describe the characteristics of a good long-term care facility.

3. Identify nursing measures to assist an older adult to meet nutritional, elimination, and personal hygiene needs.

4. List common mental health problems in older adults.

5. Explain why depression and chemical dependency are important concerns for the older person.

6. Discuss two emotional and psychological therapies and how they help the older person.

7. Explain the importance of relationships and stimulation for older adults.

8. List nursing measures to assist an older person to meet communication needs.

9. State nursing measures to assist an older person to compensate for impaired proprioception.

10. Discuss elder abuse, stating warning signs and methods of prevention.

11. Define the term *vulnerable adult*.

NEW TERMINOLOGY

aphasia	kyphosis
aspiration	presbycusis
caregiver stress	presbyopia
edentulous	proprioception
elder abuse	pseudodementia
friable	respite
geriatrics	Sjögren's syndrome
gerontology	vulnerable adult
halitosis	

KEY POINTS

- The normal aging process does not cause specific illnesses; however, lifestyle adjustments are necessary to compensate for physical changes.
- Most seniors live at home. Some older adults live in special adapted living situations.
- Many health problems in older adults relate directly or indirectly to nutrition.
- Older adults may need adjustments to basic personal hygiene measures. Skin care, nail and foot care, and adapted clothing are areas of special concern.
- Appropriate preventive care for constipation includes adequate fiber and fluids. Clients should avoid dependence on laxatives.
- Anatomic changes may lead to problems with continence.
- Presbyopia, presbycusis, and aphasia are three conditions that may hinder an older person's ability to communicate.
- Safety is an important consideration for older adults because of the loss of the sense of proprioception.
- Older clients must remain physically and mentally active to prevent anxiety, depression, and disorders caused by immobility.
- The nurse must report cases of suspected elder abuse.

■ Teaching–Learning Strategies

CLASSROOM

1. Ask the students to define the following terms:

aphasia	halitosis
geriatrics	edentulous
proprioception	kyphosis
aspiration	elder abuse
vulnerable	friable
gerontology	presbycusis
respite	presbyopia
caregiver stress	incontinence

Write the students' answers on the chalkboard or on an overhead transparency.

2. Ask students to compare and contrast home care, retirement complexes, senior day care, and long-term care facilities. Write the students' answers on the chalkboard or on an overhead transparency.

3. Before class, on an overhead transparency, write the following topics: nutrition, medications, water, hygiene, and elimination. During the class, ask the students to identify nursing considerations for the topics. Write the students' answers on the chalkboard or on an overhead transparency.

4. Briefly discuss how nurses can help to meet the emotional needs of the aging adult. Ask students to identify signs and symptoms of stress/anxiety, depression, and substance abuse. Write the students' answers on the chalkboard or on an overhead transparency.

5. Before class, on 3 × 5 index cards, write the following: communication, visual impairment, speech impairment, safety, physical activity and exercise, and sexuality. During the class, divide students into pairs and assign an index card to each pair. Ask the students to identify how nursing can assist aging adults to meet these special needs.

6. Show the videotape(s) *Elder Abuse: 5 Cases* (40 minutes) and *Not My Home* (45 minutes; both available from Fanlight Productions, 47 Halifax Street, Boston, MA 02130). After the videotape

presentation(s), open the class for questions and discussion.

CLINICAL

1. Assign students in pairs to visit an adult day care center or a senior citizens center. Ask the students to interview either an older adult at the center or one of the staff members about the role of the center. Ask students to share their experiences during clinical conference.

2. Assign students in a hospital or long-term care setting to care for an aging adult for the entire clinical day. Ask students to share their experiences during clinical conference.

3. Invite a mental health nurse who works with aging adults to visit the group and discuss special mental health concerns of the elderly. After the presentation, open the clinical conference for questions and discussion.

4. Assign students in the learning laboratory to view the series of videotapes *Normal Aging: Strategies for Optimal Health and Promoting Self Care* (1989; 6 videotapes; 30 minutes; ISBN 0-397-55878-3; available from Lippincott Williams & Wilkins, 530 Walnut Street, Philadelphia, PA 19106). Discuss the students' observations during clinical conference.

5. Before the clinical experience, ask students to research the process of reporting elder abuse in their local community. Ask students to share their findings with the larger group.

CHAPTER 92

Dementias and Related Disorders

LEARNING OBJECTIVES

1. Differentiate between confusion, delirium, and dementia.

2. List components of dementia as defined in the DSM-IV classification.

3. Describe Alzheimer's disease, its physiologic changes, and theories about its cause.

4. Identify the stages of Alzheimer's disease with accompanying common behaviors. State at least four nursing considerations for each stage.

5. Name at least two common medications used to treat Alzheimer's disease and two common adverse reactions to the medications.

6. Explain why all medication must be used with caution in older adults.

7. Identify how multi-infarct dementia differs from Alzheimer's disease.

8. Describe common methods used to diagnose dementias.

9. Discuss functional assessment of the person with dementia.

10. Apply the nursing process as it relates to clients with dementia.

NEW TERMINOLOGY

ambiguous loss	dementia
apraxia	organic brain syndrome
balking	paranoia
catastrophic reaction	pseudodementia
confabulation	respite care
confusion	senility
delirium	

Acronyms

AD	MRI
ALT	PET
CJD	SDAT
HD	SGPT
MID	SPECT

KEY POINTS

- Many reversible causes of confusion and delirium exist, including physical illness, metabolic disturbances, drug or alcohol toxicity, malnutrition, and sensory deprivation.
- Although confusion can occur at any age, the older adult is more vulnerable because of decreased physiologic reserve and the number of medications taken.
- Dementias affect the brain and nerve cells. They include Alzheimer's disease, multi-infarct dementia, Parkinson's disease, Wernicke-Korsakoff syndrome, Pick's disease, Creutzfeldt-Jakob disease, AIDS dementia, Huntington's disease, and crack-related dementia.
- Diagnosis of dementia often IS difficult; usually only brain tissue biopsy or autopsy can confirm the diagnosis. Other tests are helpful in ruling out treatable causes of dementia.
- Alzheimer's disease develops in stages, beginning with memory difficulty and progressing to increasing difficulties with memory, language, and movement. In the final stage, the client is no longer able to perform daily activities.
- Treatment for Alzheimer's is palliative; there is no known cure.
- Nursing assessment of physical and mental abilities, needs, and resources is integral in the treatment of dementia.
- One nursing goal is assessment of the client's abilities in performing basic and complex activities of daily living.

- Nursing actions when caring for the demented client include assisting with ADL, communication, and managing difficult behaviors.
- The family or caregivers of the demented client require assessment of their needs, assistance with education and respite care, and referrals to support groups.

■ Teaching–Learning Strategies

CLASSROOM

1. Ask the students to define the following terms:

advance directive
catastrophic reaction
delirium
ambiguous loss
dementia
organic brain syndrome

confabulation
aphasia
apraxia
pseudodementia
senility

Write the students' answers on the chalkboard or on an overhead transparency.

2. Show one or more of the following videotape(s) in class: *Alzheimer's Disease* (28 minutes), *Someone I Love Has Alzheimer's Disease* (17 minutes), *Something Should be Done About* *Grandma Ruthie* (54 minutes), or *Caring...Sharing: The Alzheimer's Caregiver* (all available from Fanlight Productions, 47 Halifax Street, Boston, MA 02130). After the videotape presentation(s), open the class for questions and discussion. Ask students to share their own experiences with someone they knew who had a diagnosis of Alzheimer's disease.

3. Ask students to compare and contrast confusion, delirium, and dementia. Write the student's responses on the chalkboard or on an overhead transparency.

4. Invite a mental health nurse who cares for clients with dementias and related disorders to visit the class and present the role of the nurse in caring for such clients. After the presentation, open the class for questions and discussion.

5. Show the videotape *Recognizing Delirium in the Elder Person* (1995; 30 minutes; ISBN: 0-7817-1351-X; available from Lippincott Williams & Wilkins, 530 Walnut Street, Philadelphia, PA 19106). After the videotape presentation, open the class for questions and discussion. Briefly discuss the diagnostic tests used to diagnose dementia and related disorders.

CHAPTER 93

Psychiatric Nursing

LEARNING OBJECTIVES

1. Define the most important terms and acronyms relating to mental health and its deviations.

2. Explain the normal role of defense mechanisms. Describe the results when defense mechanisms are overused.

3. Differentiate between functional and organic mental illnesses.

4. List at least five organic causes of mental illness.

5. Describe the role of neuropsychological and neurodiagnostic testing in diagnosing mental illness.

6. List at least five general symptoms of a mental disorder.

7. Describe the diagnostic criteria for a mood disorder.

8. Explain the differences between a major depressive episode and dysthymia.

9. Describe the behavioral characteristics of the person with bipolar disorder.

10. List and describe at least four personality disorders. Describe in detail common behaviors of the person with borderline personality disorder.

11. Define psychosis and list its most common symptoms.

12. Describe the relationships between substance abuse and mental illness.

13. Identify key members of the mental healthcare team and describe their roles.

14. Describe outpatient services commonly available for people with mental illnesses.

15. Identify at least three types of structured living available to clients with mental illnesses.

16. Discuss the legal categories of admission to the acute mental health setting.

17. Discuss therapies available to clients with mental illness.

18. Describe electroconvulsive therapy, indications for its use, and associated nursing implications.

19. Identify the most commonly used classifications of medications in psychiatry. Give at least three examples of each classification. Describe the undesirable side effects of neuroleptic therapy.

20. Discuss the legal rights of clients with mental illness.

21. Target approaches for dealing with aggressive or assaultive persons.

22. State the people most likely to attempt suicide and describe suicide precautions in the acute mental health setting.

23. Discuss nursing responsibilities when working with each of the following: overactive, withdrawn, depressed, hypomanic, regressive, or self-injuring clients.

NEW TERMINOLOGY

affect	defense mechanism
agoraphobia	delusion
akathisia	dual diagnosis
anhedonia	dyskinesia
anxiety	dysthymia
assaultive	dystonia
athetoid	echolalia
benzodiazepine	echopraxia
bipolar disorder	entitled
catalepsy	euthymia
catatonia	extrapyramidal
cogwheeling movement	forensic
commitment	functional disorder
compulsion	grandiosity
cyclothymic	hallucination
decanoate	

hyperinsomnia	orthostatic hypotension
hypomania	paranoid
intrusive	perseverate
lability	phobia
malingering	polydipsic
mania	psychiatric
milieu	psychometric
milieu therapy	psychosis
mood	psychotropic
mutism	rapport
neologism	regression
neuroleptic	sally port
neuroleptic malignant	schizophrenia
obsession	self-esteem
oculogyric crisis	tardive dyskinesia
opisthotonos	vulnerable adult
organic disorder	zydis

KEY POINTS

- Today, most mentally ill people are treated in the community.
- Everyone uses defense mechanisms. When they are used to extreme, a deviation from mental health exists.
- Several organic causes of mental illness exist. If healthcare professionals can locate such a cause, they can more successfully treat the illness.
- Neurologic and neuropsychological tests help to establish the diagnosis of mental illness and help to determine the plan for treatment.
- One of the most common mood disorders is major depressive episode, which is a major contributor to the act of suicide.
- The person with bipolar disorder has mood swings, from mania to depression.
- Providing care to clients with personality disorders may be very difficult.
- A psychosis is a thought disorder, with major deviations from normal behavior and lack of contact with reality. Hallucinations, delusions, and paranoia are common symptoms.
- Many mentally ill people are also chemically dependent. The two conditions complicate and contribute to one another.
- Outpatient and emergency services are available to serve clients with mental illness. Such services include a variety of structured and less-structured living situations.
- Clients may come into the healthcare facility voluntarily or may be brought in under one of several legal categories.
- Electroconvulsive therapy is used in some cases of intractable depression or when medication is contraindicated. Nurses are responsible for monitoring the client before and after the treatment and for evaluating any loss of short-term memory or cognitive changes.
- People receiving treatment for mental illness have the same rights as all other clients. Sometimes, a court order may be required to force treatment.
- Many medications that treat mental illness have unpleasant side effects. Some side effects are life threatening.
- Many psychiatric clients who use their medication are able to live productively in the community.
- Nurses must be careful with the use of patient safety devices to avoid injuring clients.
- Most clients on the mental health unit are legally considered vulnerable adults.
- It is illegal and unethical for the nurse to have social contact with vulnerable clients outside of the healthcare facility.

■ Teaching–Learning Strategies

CLASSROOM

1. Ask students to define the following terms and abbreviations:

affect	phobia
schizoid	depression
oculogyric crisis	labile
akathisia	mania
echopraxia	milieu
opisthotonos	benzodiazepine
anhedonia	compulsion
anxiety	psychotropic
euthymia	psychosis
extrapyramidal	obsession
organic disorder	delusion
athetoid	mutism
ECT	regression
paranoid	psychiatrist
mood disorder	schizophrenia
hallucination	dyskinesia
dual diagnosis	dystonia
catalepsy	bipolar disorder (BPD)
intrusive	

Write the students' responses on the chalkboard or on an overhead transparency.

2. During class, ask students to identify symptoms of mental illness. Write the students' responses on the chalkboard or on an overhead transparency.

3. Before class, using 3 × 5 index cards, write the following topics: mood disorders, personality disorders, anxiety disorders, psychosis, and dual diagnosis. During the class, divide students into pairs and assign each pair one of the index cards. Ask students to outline the disorder and provide examples. Ask students to share their findings with the larger group.

4. Briefly discuss the types of admissions to an inpatient psychiatric unit. Discuss types of psychiatric therapy and ask the students to contrast the different therapies.

5. Before class, using 3 × 5 index cards, write numerous key medications used in psychiatric therapies. Assign students to research one or more of these drugs and present their findings to the larger group. Students should include normal dosages, use, and any significant notes about the drug.

6. Ask a nurse employed in a psychiatric inpatient setting to visit the class and discuss nursing care of mentally ill clients. After the presentation, open the class for questions and discussion.

CLINICAL

1. Assign students to care for a client in an inpatient psychiatric setting. After the clinical experience, ask students to share their experiences during clinical conference.

2. Assign students to observe in an outpatient mental health clinic. Ask students to interview a nurse in the clinic about the types of services offered. After the clinical experience, ask students to share their experiences during clinical conference.

3. Ask students to design a poster related to prevention of stress-related illnesses. Have the students bring the posters to clinical conference. Offer to donate the students' posters to a mental health clinic.

4. Before the clinical experience, ask pairs of students to identify community mental health services. Ask the students to share their findings during clinical conference.

CHAPTER 94

Substance Abuse

LEARNING OBJECTIVES

1. List the criteria for a diagnosis of substance abuse and of chemical dependency.

2. Discuss possible contributing factors to development of chemical dependency.

3. List specific steps in managing various types of chemical dependency.

4. Describe signs that you might see in a client that indicate substance abuse, including characteristic behavior changes and physical signs.

5. Identify components of nursing assessment for chemical dependency.

6. Describe nursing measures in detoxification.

7. Explain the term *refeeding syndrome*.

8. Identify methods for the long-term treatment of chemical dependency.

9. List stages of alcohol withdrawal.

10. Describe the specific nursing care in alcohol withdrawal.

11. Describe the role of the co-dependent in alcoholism.

12. List the signs of abuse and withdrawal symptoms for drugs other than alcohol.

13. Explain how opiate-blocker drugs are used in maintenance programs for narcotic substance abuse.

14. Discuss the danger of the abuse of hallucinogens and volatile substances.

15. Discuss concepts related to the abuse of anabolic steroids, nicotine, and caffeine.

16. Describe problems related to the abuse of over-the-counter drugs.

17. Identify special problems associated with drug abuse in pregnant women, adolescents, and older adults.

18. Discuss legal obligations of nurses who believe co-workers are abusing drugs or alcohol.

NEW TERMINOLOGY

agonist therapy	macropsia
alcohol hallucinosis	micropsia
aversion therapy	nystagmus
blackout	polysubstance abuse
chemical/substance	refeeding syndrome
abuse	remission
chemical/substance	rhinorrhea
dependence	substance abuse
cirrhosis	tolerance
co-dependent	Wernicke-Korsakoff
delirium tremens	syndrome
detoxification	withdrawal
dual disorder	
enabler	

Acronyms

AA	$MgSO_4$
ACOA	MI/CD
APA	MJ
ARLD	MVA
ASI	NA
CD	NSAID
DIS	OBS
DTs	OTC
DUI/DWI	PCP
ETOH	RET/REBT
FAS	STP
LSD	THC
MADD	W/D
MDA/MDMA	WKS

KEY POINTS

- Substance abuse and chemical dependency are serious public health problems that cost millions of dollars and take many lives yearly.
- Major precipitating factors of chemical abuse include stress and low self-esteem.
- The person with a dual disorder, such as mental illness and chemical dependency, may experience more difficulty in achieving a successful recovery.
- Management of substance abuse involves recognition, intervention, treatment, and recovery.
- Clients admitted to any healthcare facility may be substance abusers. Watch for withdrawal symptoms in all clients. Do not assume that any client is exempt from the possibility of chemical abuse.
- Care of a client during detoxification requires excellent assessment and nursing skills.
- Detoxification differs, depending on the abused drug and other physical and emotional factors.
- Certain blocker or agonist medications may be used as adjunct treatment for long-term management of chronic, intractable chemical dependency.
- Most clients require long-term follow-up and after-care after detoxification and intensive chemical dependency treatment.
- The co-dependent or enabler is a key figure in alcoholism.
- Substance abuse is an especially serious problem for selected groups, including pregnant women, adolescents, and older adults.
- Nurses are more likely to abuse substances than are members of the general population.

■ Teaching–Learning Strategies

CLASSROOM

1. Ask students to identify the following terms:

agonist therapy	chemical dependency
co-dependent	nystagmus
refeeding syndrome	tolerance
delirium tremens	withdrawal
aversion therapy	polysubstance abuse
detoxification	addictions
blackouts	recovery
enabler	

Write the students' answers on the chalkboard or on an overhead transparency.

2. Show the videotape *The Substance in Question* (36 minutes) or *Teens and Alcoholism* (18 minutes; both available from Films for the Humanities and Sciences, P.O. Box 2053, Princeton, NJ 08543). After the videotape presentation(s), open the class for questions and discussion.

3. Ask students to identify the causes, nature, and care of clients with substance abuse problems. List the students' responses on the chalkboard or on an overhead transparency.

4. Divide students into pairs. Ask students to design a nursing care plan for a client undergoing withdrawal symptoms. Ask the students to share their care plans with the larger group.

5. Briefly discuss abuse of substances other than alcohol. Show the videotape *Cocaine: The End of the Line* (58 minutes; available from Films for the Humanities and Sciences, P.O. Box 2053, Princeton, NJ 08543). After the videotape presentation, open the class for questions and discussion.

6. Invite a nurse who cares for clients with substance abuse problems and ask the nurse to present the role of the nurse in caring for these clients. After the presentation, open the class for questions and discussion.

7. Show the videotape *Impaired Nursing Practice: Assessment and Intervention* (1988; 28 minutes; available from Lippincott Williams & Wilkins, 530 Walnut Street, Philadelphia, PA 19106). After the videotape presentation, discuss the implications of substance abuse in co-workers.

CLINICAL

1. Arrange for pairs of students to attend a self-help group for clients experiencing substance abuse problems. Ask students to share their experiences during clinical conference.

2. Ask students to research available treatment centers for substance abuse clients in their local community. Ask students to share their findings with the larger group.

3. Assign small groups of students to care for substance abuse clients in an inpatient clinical setting. Ask the students to observe during a group therapy session. Ask students to share their observations with the larger group.

4. Ask each student to interview an adolescent about substance abuse in adolescents. Have each student write a brief one- to two-page report and present the report during clinical conference.

5. Assign a small group of students to an outpatient clinic that treats special cases of substance abuse, such as pregnant women. After the experience, ask students to share their observations with the larger group.

SUGGESTED RESOURCES: VIDEOTAPES

Autism. (1992). [28 minutes]. Available from Aquarius Health Care Videos, P.O. Box 1159, Sherborn, MA 01770)

Back from madness: The struggle for sanity. [53 minutes]. (Available from Films for the Humanities and Sciences, P.O. Box 2053, Princeton, NJ 08543-2053)

Depression and manic depression. (1996). [28 minutes]. (Available from Aquarius Health Care Videos, P.O. Box 1159, Sherborn, MA 01770)

Depression in the long term care setting. (1992). [28 minutes]. (Available from Lippincott Williams & Wilkins, 530 Walnut Street, Philadelphia, PA 19106)

Inside schizophrenia. (1997). [33 minutes]. (Available from Aquarius Health Care Videos, P.O. Box 1159, Sherborn, MA 01770)

Mental illness. [23 minutes]. (Available from Films for the Humanities and Sciences, P.O. Box 2053, Princeton, NJ 08543-2053)

Schizophrenia. [20 minutes]. (Available from Films for the Humanities and Sciences, P.O. Box 2053, Princeton, NJ 08543-2053)

ADDITIONAL RESOURCES:

Adult Children of Alcoholics, World Service Organization, telephone: 310-534-1815

Al-Anon Family Group Headquarters and Al-A-Teen, telephone: 757-563-1600

Alcoholics Anonymous World Services, General Service Office, telephone: 212-870-3400

Alternative Medicine Foundation, HerbMed, website: *www.herbmed.org*

Cocaine Anonymous, World Service Office, telephone: 310-559-5833; hotline: 310-216-4444

CODA (Co-Dependents Anonymous), telephone: 602-277-7991

Hazelden, telephone: 800-328-9000; website: *www.hazelden.org*

Narcotics Anonymous, World Service Office, telephone: 818-773-9999

National Al-Anon Hotline, telephone: 800-344-2666 (messages in English, Spanish, and French)

National Clearinghouse for Alcohol and Drug Abuse Information, P.O. Box 2345, 11400 Rockville Pike, Rockville, MD 20852; telephone: 800-729-6686 (messages in English and Spanish)

Nicotine Anonymous, World Service Office, telephone: 415-750-0328; website: *www.nicotine-anonymous.org*

Sex Addicts Anonymous, International Service Organization, telephone: 713-869-4902

Workaholics Anonymous, World Service Organization, telephone: 510-273-9253

CHAPTER 95

Extended Care

LEARNING OBJECTIVES

1. Describe the continuum of healthcare from acute care to independent living.

2. Differentiate between the major types of long-term facilities.

3. Describe and discuss the concept of transitional facilities.

4. List community resources available to persons living in their own homes.

5. Identify optional services or amenities that may be available at an extended care facility.

NEW TERMINOLOGY

assisted living	ombudsman
congregate housing	subacute care
medically complex nursing unit	vulnerable adult payee

KEY POINTS

- Many lifestyle options are available for people who need varying levels of assistance.
- Clients may move from one type of lifestyle option to another as their needs change.
- The least restrictive type of care should be given to promote the client's independent functioning.
- The vast majority of older adults and people with physical and mental challenges live independently.
- Today's long-term care facilities offer safe and comfortable living. Many offer a wide variety of amenities.

■ Teaching–Learning Strategies

CLASSROOM

1. Ask students to define the following terms and abbreviations:

   assisted living
   intermediate care facilities
   congregate housing
   medically complex nursing unit
   ombudsman
   skilled nursing facility
   subacute care
   unlicensed assistive personnel
   vulnerable adult

   Write the students' responses on the chalkboard or on an overhead transparency.

2. Ask the students to share their personal experiences with extended care facilities. Outline the students' responses on the chalkboard or on an overhead transparency.

3. Ask the students to compare and contrast the various types of short-term and long-term care facilities. Outline the students' responses on the chalkboard or on an overhead transparency.

4. Invite a nurse or other health professional who is employed by a short-term or long-term care facility to address the class on his or her role in these facilities. After the presentation, open the class for questions and discussion.

CLINICAL

1. Arrange for pairs of students to observe a nurse in a short-term or long-term care facility. Ask the students to share their observations with the larger group.

2. Arrange for small groups of students to care for clients in a short-term or long-term care facility. Ask the students to share their nursing care plans for the client with the larger group.

CHAPTER 96

Rehabilitation Nursing

LEARNING OBJECTIVES

1. Explain the goals of rehabilitation.

2. Describe the stages of adjustment to disabling illness or injury.

3. Identify members of the rehabilitation team and their roles.

4. Relate rehabilitation to Maslow's hierarchy of needs.

5. Differentiate between functional and instrumental activities of daily living (ADL).

6. Explain adaptive equipment and home modifications that assist clients to independently perform ADLs.

7. Describe rehabilitation in terms of mobility.

8. Discuss the major elements of a continence program.

9. Describe general rehabilitation for people with disabling musculoskeletal, cardiovascular, or neurologic disorders.

10. Give examples of community resources for people with physical and mental challenges.

11. Define the term *architectural barrier* and identify several in your community.

12. Identify barriers to rehabilitation for individuals and communities.

NEW TERMINOLOGY

architectural barriers	paraplegic
exoskeleton	physiatrist
hemiplegic	prosthetics
mainstreaming	quadriplegic
neurogenic	rehabilitation
orthotics	

Acronyms

ALS	CVA
CF	FADL
FES	MS
HD	PPS
IADL	PM&R
MD	TBI

KEY POINTS

- Rehabilitation aims to restore a person to full functioning or to maximize the client's remaining abilities.
- Professionals from many different disciplines function as a part of the rehabilitation team.
- The client and the primary caregivers are vital members of the rehabilitation team.
- Clients and families often work through predictable stages of grief in dealing with serious illness or disabling injury.
- Rehabilitation team members assist clients in performing strengthening exercises to prevent falls or other injury and to provide mobility.
- Adaptive materials are available to assist the person with a disability to perform ADL.
- Many pieces of equipment, including wheelchairs, scooters, walkers, splints, and braces help provide mobility to people with disabilities.
- Continence management is a major component of rehabilitation.
- Many community resources are available to assist people who have disabilities or chronic conditions and their families.

■Teaching–Learning Strategies

CLASSROOM

1. Ask students to define the following terms and abbreviations:

   architectural   orthotics
     barriers   hemiplegic
   quadriplegic   physiatrist
   mainstreaming   prosthetics
   neurogenic   functional ADLs
   exoskeleton   instrumental ADLs

   Write the students' responses on the chalkboard or on an overhead transparency.

2. Ask the students to share their personal experiences with rehabilitation services. Outline the students' responses on the chalkboard or on an overhead transparency.

3. Invite a nurse or other health professional who is employed in rehabilitative services to address the class regarding the nurse's role in these facilities. After the presentation, open the class for questions and discussion.

CLINICAL

1. Arrange for small groups of students to visit various rehabilitative facilities for an entire clinical day. Ask the students to share their observations with the larger group.

CHAPTER 97

Ambulatory Nursing

LEARNING OBJECTIVES

1. Explain what is meant by the "trend toward community-based healthcare delivery."

2. Describe the functions of the nurse who works in a physician's office, in an emergency room or urgent care center, and in a same-day surgery center.

3. Discuss the benefits of same-day surgery.

4. Describe scientific developments that have made same-day surgery possible.

5. List and describe the classifications of potential clients for same-day surgery.

6. Describe the importance of client and family teaching in ambulatory healthcare.

NEW TERMINOLOGY

cardioversion	port
emergi-center	stabilization (sta-be) room
endoscopy	telehealth
managed care protocol	vertical clients

Acronyms

ACS	FHC
CHC	HMO
CIC, crisis intervention center	PCP
	SRO
EHS	

KEY POINTS

- Ambulatory nursing care may be delivered in a physician's office or clinic, urgent care center, community health center, day surgery, or in the client's home.
- Nurses function as direct assistants to physicians in many ambulatory care settings.
- Nurses who work in ambulatory settings need multiple skills. They may require additional training to perform some skills.

- The family/community health center provides primary care and secondary services for many people. These centers employ large numbers of nurses.
- Clients coming in for same-day surgery or in the morning for inpatient surgery need a great deal of instruction because most preoperative preparation is done at home.
- Same-day surgery clients and many clients discharged soon after surgery (as well as their primary caregivers) need follow-up care after discharge to ensure proper recovery.
- Documentation is vital in all phases of ambulatory care, as it is in inpatient settings.

■Teaching–Learning Strategies

CLASSROOM

1. Ask students to define the following terms:

   crisis intervention center
   emergi-center
   cardioversion
   port
   community/family health center
   telehealth
   vertical clients
   same-day surgery center
   endoscopy
   stabilization room

   Write the students' responses on the chalkboard or on an overhead transparency.

2. Ask a nurse who is employed in an ambulatory care center to visit the class and discuss the topic of the nurse's role in these care settings. After the presentation, open the class for discussion and questions.

3. Ask the students to share their personal experiences with ambulatory care.

CLINICAL

1. Arrange for pairs of students to observe a nurse in an ambulatory care setting. Ask the students to interview the nurse about his or her role in working with clients. Ask the students to share their experiences with the larger group.

2. Arrange for pairs of students to observe in a day surgery center. Ask the students to write a one- to two-page paper describing their experiences and share with the larger group.

CHAPTER 98

Home Care Nursing

LEARNING OBJECTIVES

1. Identify the reasons for and the benefits of home care.

2. Describe situations in which home care might be most appropriate.

3. Identify several nursing functions in home care.

4. Discuss important safety practices for home care nurses.

5. Describe and discuss the influences of regulatory agencies upon delivery of home healthcare.

6. Describe recent changes in reimbursement for home care.

NEW TERMINOLOGY

Acronyms

CNO	NAHC
(C)HHA	OASIS
HCA	PCA
HHRG	PPS

KEY POINTS

- The community health center and home care nursing are the fastest growing segments of the healthcare delivery system.
- Clients are being discharged from acute care facilities with complex nursing needs, which home care workers and family caregivers must meet.
- Home care nurses have the opportunity to schedule hours and to structure their own time.
- Home care nurses must be alert to untoward signs and symptoms and report them to the appropriate person.

- Many clients opt for home care because it is cost effective and often more comfortable than hospital care.
- Home care nurses are ultimately responsible for their own personal safety.

■ Teaching–Learning Strategies

CLASSROOM

1. Show the videotape *Home Care Nursing Visit Procedures: The Initial Visit* (22 minutes; available from Lippincott Williams & Wilkins, 530 Walnut Street, Philadelphia, PA 19106). After the videotape presentation, open the class for discussion.

2. Ask a nurse who is employed in a home care center to visit the class and discuss the topic of the nurse's role in these care settings. After the presentation, open the class for discussion and questions.

3. Ask the students to share their personal experiences with home care.

CLINICAL

1. Arrange for the students to make home care visits with a nurse. After the experience, ask the students to share their experiences with the larger group.

2. Ask pairs of students to research the local community services available that provide health care assistance. Ask the students to share their findings with the larger group.

CHAPTER 99

Hospice Nursing

LEARNING OBJECTIVES

1. Discuss the evolution of the hospice movement.

2. Name the four areas of human needs on which the hospice concept focuses.

3. List at least six characteristics a program must meet to be officially classified as a hospice.

4. Explain the criteria for a person's admission to a hospice program

5. Define the term *respite care* and explain the purpose of such care.

6. Define interdisciplinary care as it applies to hospice; identify the major disciplines involved.

7. Differentiate between the functions of the case manager, the hospice nurse, and other members of the healthcare team.

8. Discuss the role of primary caregivers in hospice.

9. Describe emotional and spiritual support for the client and family.

10. Identify measures used for odor management and measures used to treat anorexia, nausea and vomiting, constipation, diarrhea, respiratory distress, and skin breakdown for hospice clients.

11. Discuss threats to mental health, such as depression and anxiety, which can occur in hospice clients and caregivers.

12. Identify medications used for pain management in hospice.

13. List and briefly describe three psychosocial modalities used for pain management.

14. List and describe at least two physical modalities used in pain management.

15. Discuss important considerations when caring for children in hospice programs.

16. Explain the nurse's role after the client dies.

NEW TERMINOLOGY

ablative surgery	palliative care
adjuvant	primary caregivers
bereavement	respite
debulking	somnolent
hospice	titration
interdisciplinary care	

Acronyms

BSC	MSW
CRNH	NYPCO
COPs	OBT
DME	PCA
DNH	POC
DNI	PSDA
DNR	SI
IDG	TENS
IDT	

KEY POINTS

- Hospice care is designed for terminally ill people. Its focus is providing aggressive, intensive palliative care and assisting with physical, psychological, social, and spiritual needs.
- The client is assisted toward self-actualization, as much as is possible.
- Respite care may be necessary for family members.
- Several disciplines work together with clients and families to deliver compassionate end-of-life care.
- Hospice programs provide follow-up care to families for 1 year after a loved one's death, to assist with bereavement. They encourage support group membership.
- Education of family caregivers is a major hospice nursing goal.
- The goal of pain and symptom management is relief without unwanted side effects.
- Hospice care is very difficult. Clients and caregivers can experience deviations from mental health, such as depression and anxiety.
- The nurse and family caregivers work together to perform final care and make final preparations after the client dies.

- Hospice staff members also need assistance and support to help them deal with the emotional stress of continuously working with dying people and their families.

▪ Teaching–Learning Strategies

CLASSROOM

1. Ask the students to define the following terms and abbreviations:

ablative surgery	adjuvant
palliative care	bereavement
hospice	titration
somnolent	anorexia
NSAIDs	debulking
primary caregivers	analgesic ladder

Write the students' responses on the chalkboard or on an overhead transparency.

2. Ask the students to identify the roles of each of the following involved in hospice care: nurse, primary caregiver, physician, volunteer, social services, and bereavement counselor. Write the students' responses on the chalkboard or on an overhead transparency.

3. Ask a nurse or volunteer who works with hospice clients to visit the class and describe the types of clients cared for and their roles. After the presentation, open the class for questions and discussion.

4. Show the videotape *Companions on a Journey* (1997; 22 minutes; available from Aquarius Productions, Inc., P.O. Box 1159, Sherborn, MA 01770; *www.aquariusproductions.com*). After the videotape presentation, open the class for questions and discussion.

5. Ask students to share their personal experiences with terminally ill family members or hospice care.

CLINICAL

1. Arrange for pairs of students to visit a hospice unit. After the experience, ask students to share their observations with the larger group.

2. Ask the students to use the Internet or library to locate articles related to hospice care. Ask the students to write a one-page summary of the article and share their findings with the larger group.

3. In the clinical setting, arrange for as many students as possible to join a nurse to care for clients who are considered terminally ill. Ask the students to share their feelings about the experience during clinical conference.

SUGGESTED RESOURCES: VIDEOTAPES

Aging well. [16 minutes]. (Available from Films for the Humanities and Sciences, P.O. Box 2053, Princeton, NJ 08543-2053)

Chronic anxiety in the elderly. [28 minutes]. (Available from Films for the Humanities and Sciences, P.O. Box 2053, Princeton, NJ 08543-2053)

Hospice care: A positive choice. [7 minutes]. (Available from Lippincott Williams & Wilkins, 530 Walnut Street, Philadelphia, PA 19106)

Living wills. (1992). [29 minutes]. (Available from Aquarius Productions, Inc., P.O. Box 1159, Sherborn, MA 01770)

A matter of time. (1996). [20 minutes]. (Available from Aquarius Productions, Inc., P.O. Box 1159, Sherborn, MA 01770)

On life and living: The hospice experience. (1993). [18 minutes]. (Available from Aquarius Productions, Inc., P.O. Box 1159, Sherborn, MA 01770)

Pneumonia in the long term setting. (1992). [30 minutes]. (Available from Lippincott Williams & Wilkins, 530 Walnut Street, Philadelphia, PA 19106)

We can do it: Children cope with cancer. (1991). [14 minutes]. (Available from Lippincott Williams & Wilkins, 530 Walnut Street, Philadelphia, PA 19106)

CHAPTER 100

From Student to Graduate Nurse

LEARNING OBJECTIVES

1. Describe the importance of obtaining a license to practice nursing.

2. Explain how the NCLEX examination relates to the steps of the nursing process.

3. Define the categories of client needs measured by the NCLEX examination.

4. List at least four just causes for which a nurse's license may be revoked or suspended.

5. Identify at least six entry-level competencies expected of an LPN/LVN.

6. Describe the value of the Internet for a graduate nurse.

7. Discuss at least four differences in activities or client behavior that may occur during evening or night shifts, as opposed to daytime hours.

8. Describe at least five ways in which a nurse can protect his or her health while working the night shift.

9. Identify the components of a personal nursing file.

NEW TERMINOLOGY

career mobility
Internet
transcribing orders

KEY POINTS

- Nurses must pass the NCLEX examination to obtain nursing licensure and to practice nursing.
- The NCLEX examination, a computer adaptive test rather than a paper-and-pencil test, is based on a job analysis of tasks that actual nurses perform in the course of their employment.
- Most states require renewal of a nursing license every 1 or 2 years, along with evidence of continuing education.

- After becoming licensed, a nurse may wish to move and transfer his or her licensure to another state.
- Entry-level skills of the LPN/LVN include data collection, planning, implementation, evaluation, member of the discipline, managing/supervising, and political activism.
- Maintaining client confidentiality, organizing workload, taking and transcribing orders, using technology, and maintaining a current knowledge base are important for the graduate LPN/LVN.
- Nurses are responsible for continuity of client care 24 hours a day; the atmosphere and some activities in the healthcare facility during the evening and night hours may differ from those of day hours.
- A graduate nurse is responsible for keeping up with current trends in nursing. By being an active member of a nursing organization, a graduate nurse will be able to keep in touch with new advancements in nursing and with current trends.
- The graduate nurse must learn to balance the demands of work with his or her personal responsibilities and activities.

■ Teaching–Learning Strategies

CLASSROOM

1. Ask the student to define the following terms:

career mobility	reciprocity
transcribing	probationary
entry level skills	NCLEX-PN
Internet	

   Write the student's responses on the chalkboard or overhead transparency.

2. Invite a graduate nurse who has just sat for her NCLEX-PN boards to discuss the process with the class, including the emotional and physiological responses of the graduate nurse.

3. Have the students begin a personal file of professional information or a professional portfolio.

CLINICAL

1. In the clinical learning laboratory, have the students practice checking physician orders. Provide the student with sample charts. Role play a situation in which the physician is telephoning an order for a client in the acute care setting.

2. In the clinical setting, ask the student to practice checking physicians' orders. Ask the students to share their experiences during clinical conference.

3. In the clinical setting, have the students observe how different nurses organize their workday and routines. Have the students share this information in clinical conference.

CHAPTER 101

Career Opportunities and Job-Seeking Skills

LEARNING OBJECTIVES

1. List at least six types of healthcare facilities or related agencies in which LPNs/LVNs might seek employment, other than the hospital or long-term care facility.

2. List at least five specialized areas of nursing available to the LPN/LVN.

3. Name at least four sources of employment information for nurses.

4. Explain how a nurse might conduct a job search or apply for a position using the Internet.

5. Describe the function of a placement service, nursing pool, or registry.

6. Identify at least six important personal considerations and six professional considerations when choosing a place of employment.

7. List items to include in a résumé. Demonstrate the ability to prepare a personal résumé.

8. Describe the letter of application and procedures for filling out the application form. Demonstrate the ability to correctly complete an application for a position.

9. Describe preparation for and protocols during a job interview.

10. Identify the proper protocol for resigning from a position.

NEW TERMINOLOGY

nurse's registry
telehealth

Acronyms

EHS
HBO

KEY POINTS

- Multiple employment opportunities exist in nursing and in other healthcare fields.
- The graduate nurse can choose employment to fit his or her personal needs—different practice areas, structured or less-structured settings, self-employment, and different parts of the country or world.
- Nurses must consider their personal goals and lifestyles when choosing the "best fit" for employment.
- Completing and updating your résumé is an integral component of your job search.
- People form their first impressions in a matter of seconds; a positive first impression is important in obtaining employment.
- The personal interview offers you and the employer the opportunity to learn about each other.
- Many opportunities for continuing education are available. Many employers finance some courses.
- Your nursing license is your passport to employment. You must maintain it if you wish to work in nursing.
- Nurses should become involved in professional organizations and in their local communities.
- Keep a file of professional information so that you can retrieve necessary documents easily.
- You can conduct a job search, apply for a position, and take continuing education courses via the Internet.
- Your nursing education is just beginning. You will be learning the rest of your professional life.

■ Teaching–Learning Strategies

CLASSROOM

1. Ask the students to define the following terms:

   telehealth
   travel nurse
   nurse's registry
   résumé

   Write the students' responses on the chalkboard or on an overhead transparency.

2. Invite a nurse who is involved in interviewing or hiring LPN/LVN graduates in a local setting. Ask the nurse to discuss the topic of interviewing and hiring. After the presentation, open the class for questions and discussion.

3. During the class, ask two students to volunteer to role plan an interview scenario. Ask one of the students to play the role of the nurse who is responsible for hiring and the other to play the role of the job seeker. After the role-playing exercise, open the class for questions and discussion.

4. Before class, ask the students to use the Internet to locate employment opportunities. Ask the students to bring a hard copy of the employment opportunity to class and share their findings with the larger group.

CLINICAL

1. During the clinical laboratory, ask the students to write a résumé. Using the Internet, ask the students to locate a site that assists with résumé writing or other employment services.

2. Assign pairs of students to visit clinical settings that are different from acute care institutions or long-term care settings, such as prisons or parishes. After the experience, ask the students to share their experiences with the larger group.

SUGGESTED RESOURCES: VIDEOTAPES

Confidentiality: Legal and ethical concerns in health care. (1996). [24 minutes]. (Available from Insight Media, P.O. Box 621, New York, NY 10024)

Documenting nursing practice. (1997). [28 minutes]. (Available from Insight Media, P.O. Box 621, New York, NY 10024)

Leadership. (Available from Insight Media, P.O. Box 621, New York, NY 10024)

Time management skills. (1992). [18 minutes]. (Available from Lippincott Williams & Wilkins, 530 Walnut Street, Philadelphia, PA 19106)

Transcultural nursing: Discovery and challenge. (1992). [22 minutes]. (Available from Insight Media, P.O. Box 621, New York, NY 10024)

CHAPTER 102

Advancement and Leadership in Nursing

LEARNING OBJECTIVES

1. Describe how an LPN/LVN can become nationally certified in long-term care.

2. Compare and contrast the terms *leader* and *manager*.

3. Discuss the characteristics of a good manager.

4. Describe leadership roles available to the LPN/LVN.

5. State at least four duties of the charge nurse and team leader.

6. List at least three characteristics of an effective manager.

7. Describe four different leadership styles.

NEW TERMINOLOGY

autocratic leadership	leader
bureaucratic leadership	manager
democratic leadership	performance review
due process	plan of assistance
laissez-faire leadership	oral/written reprimand

KEY POINTS

- The role of all nurses, including LPNs, is expanding.
- LPNs can be nationally certified in long-term care.
- Many LPN/LVNs work as charge nurses or team leaders, especially in extended care facilities.
- A new graduate of a nursing program needs additional education and experience before assuming a leadership role.
- Several different leadership styles exist. There is no right or wrong style; any of them can be effective.
- Specific evaluation procedures must be followed in order to ensure due process for employees.

■ Teaching–Learning Strategies

CLASSROOM

1. Ask the students to define the following terms:

autocratic	laissez-faire
bureaucratic	certification
democratic	continuity of nursing care

   Write the students' responses on the chalkboard or on an overhead transparency.

2. Ask two students to volunteer for a role-playing situation. Assign one of the students to be the "leader" and provide the student with a scenario (e.g., delegation). Ask the "leader" to assume a particular leadership style (e.g., autocratic). After the role-playing situation, open the class for questions and discussions.

3. Conduct a discussion with the class about the differences between working on a day shift as compared to evenings or nights.

4. Invite a nurse who is certified as an LPN/LVN in long-term care to address the class on the topic of certification. Following the presentation, open the class for questions and discussions.

CLINICAL

1. Assign students to the clinical setting (one clinical experience) on the evening or night shift. Assign students to one client to provide nursing care. After the experience, ask students to share their observations with the larger group.

2. In the learning laboratory, ask the students to join a nursing "listserv" on the Internet. After a 1 week period, ask the students to share topics being discussed.

3. Assign students to the clinical setting (one clinical experience) on the evening or night shift. Assign students to one client to provide nursing care.

After the experience, ask students to share their observations with the larger group.

SUGGESTED RESOURCES: VIDEOTAPES

Leadership. (Available from Insight Media, P.O. Box 621, New York, NY 10024)

North American Nursing Diagnosis Association (NANDA) Accepted Nursing Diagnoses

Activity Intolerance
Activity Intolerance, Risk for
Acute Confusion
Acute Pain
Adaptive Capacity, Decreased Intracranial
Adjustment, Impaired
Adult Failure to Thrive
Airway Clearance, Ineffective
Alcoholism, Dysfunctional Family Responses
Allergy Responses, Latex
Allergy Responses, Latex, Risk for
Anticipatory Grieving
Anxiety
Anxiety, Death
Aspiration, Risk for
Attachment, Risk for Impaired Parent/Infant/Child
Autonomic Dysreflexia
Autonomic Dysreflexia, Risk for
Bathing/Hygiene Self-Care Deficit
Bed Mobility, Impaired
Body Image, Disturbed
Body Temperature, Risk for Imbalanced
Bowel Incontinence
Breastfeeding, Effective
Breastfeeding, Ineffective
Breastfeeding, Interrupted
Breathing Pattern, Ineffective
Cardiac Output, Decreased
Caregiver Role Strain
Caregiver Role Strain, Risk for
Chronic Confusion
Chronic Pain
Chronic Sorrow
Communication, Impaired Verbal
Compromised Family Coping
Conflict, Decisional
Conflict, Parental Role
Confusion, Acute
Confusion, Chronic
Constipation
Constipation, Perceived

Constipation, Risk for
Coping, Defensive
Coping, Ineffective
Coping, Ineffective Community
Coping, Readiness for Enhanced Community
Coping, Compromised Family
Coping, Disabled Family
Coping, Readiness for Enhanced
Death Anxiety
Decisional Conflict
Decreased Cardiac Output
Denial, Ineffective
Dentition, Impaired
Development, Risk for Delayed
Diarrhea
Disproportionate Growth, Risk for
Disturbed Body Image
Disuse Syndrome, Risk for
Diversional Activity, Deficient
Dressing/Grooming Self-Care Deficit
Dysreflexia, Autonomic
Elimination, Impaired Urinary
Energy Field, Disturbed
Environmental Interpretation Syndrome, Impaired
Excess Fluid Volume
Failure to Thrive, Adult
Falls, Risk for
Family Processes Dysfunctional: Alcoholism
Family Processes Dysfunctional: Alcoholism, Interrupted
Fatigue
Fear
Feeding Self-Care Deficit
Fluid Volume, Deficient
Fluid Volume, Excess
Fluid Volume, Risk for Deficient
Fluid Volume, Risk for Imbalanced
Gas Exchange, Impaired
Grieving, Anticipatory
Grieving, Dysfunctional
Growth and Development, Delayed

Growth, Risk for Disproportionate
Health Maintenance, Ineffective
Home Maintenance, Impaired
Hopelessness
Hyperthermia
Hypothermia
Identity, Disturbed Personal
Imbalanced Fluid Volume, Risk for
Incontinence, Bowel
Incontinence, Functional Urinary
Incontinence, Reflex Urinary
Incontinence, Stress Urinary
Incontinence, Total Urinary
Incontinence, Urge Urinary
Incontinence, Risk for Urge Urinary
Infant Behavior, Disorganized
Infant Behavior, Readiness for Enhanced
Infant Behavior, Organized
Infant Feeding Pattern, Ineffective
Infection, Risk for
Injury, Risk for Perioperative-Positioning
Injury, Risk for
Intracranial Adaptive Capacity, Decreased
Interrupted Breastfeeding
Knowledge, Deficient
Latex Allergy Response, Risk for
Loneliness, Risk for
Memory, Impaired
Mobility, Impaired Bed
Mobility, Impaired Physical
Mobility, Impaired Wheelchair
Mucous Membrane, Impaired Oral
Nausea
Neglect, Unilateral
Neurovascular Dysfunction, Risk for Peripheral
Noncompliance
Nutrition, Imbalanced: Less Than Body
   Requirements
Nutrition, Imbalanced: More Than Body
   Requirements
Nutrition, Risk for Imbalanced: More Than body
   Requirements
Oral Mucous Membrane, Impaired
Organized Infant Behavior, Readiness for Enhanced
Pain, Acute
Pain, Chronic
Parental Role Conflict
Parent/Infant/Child Attachment, Risk for Impaired
Parenting, Impaired
Parenting, Impaired, Risk for
Perceived Constipation
Perioperative-Positioning Injury, Risk for
Peripheral Neurovascular Dysfunction, Risk for
Personal Identity, Disturbed
Physical Mobility, Impaired

Poisoning, Risk for
Post-Trauma Syndrome
Post-Trauma Syndrome, Risk for
Powerlessness
Powerlessness, Risk for
Protection, Ineffective
Rape-Trauma Syndrome
Rape-Trauma Syndrome, Compound Reaction
Rape-Trauma Syndrome, Silent Reaction
Recovery, Delayed Surgical
Relocation Stress Syndrome
Relocation Stress Syndrome, Risk for
Retention, Urinary
Role Conflict, Parental
Role Performance, Ineffective
Role Strain, Caregiver
Role Strain, Caregiver, Risk for
Self-Care Deficit, Bathing/Hygiene
Self-Care Deficit, Dressing/Grooming
Self-Care Deficit, Feeding
Self-Care Deficit, Toileting
Self-Esteem, Low
Self-Esteem, Chronic Low
Self-Esteem, Situational Low
Self-Esteem, Risk for Situational Low
Self-Mutilation
Self-Mutilation, Risk for
Sensory Perception, Disturbed
Sexual Dysfunction
Sexuality Patterns, Ineffective
Skin Integrity, Impaired
Skin Integrity, Impaired, Risk for
Sleep Deprivation
Sleep Pattern, Disturbed
Social Interaction, Impaired
Social Isolation
Sorrow, Chronic
Spiritual Distress
Spiritual Distress, Risk for
Spiritual Well-Being, Readiness for Enhanced
Suffocation, Risk for
Suicide, Risk for
Surgical Recovery, Delayed
Swallowing, Impaired
Syndrome, Risk for Disuse
Syndrome, Impaired Environmental Interpretation
Syndrome, Post-Trauma
Syndrome, Risk for Post-Trauma
Syndrome, Rape-Trauma
Syndrome, Compound Reaction Rape-Trauma
Syndrome, Silent Reaction Rape-Trauma
Therapeutic Regimen Management, Effective
Therapeutic Regimen Management, Ineffective
Therapeutic Regimen Management, Ineffective
   Community

Therapeutic Regimen Management, Ineffective
   Family
Thermoregulation, Ineffective
Thought Processes, Disturbed
Tissue Integrity, Impaired
Tissue Perfusion, Ineffective
Toileting Self-Care Deficit
Transfer Ability, Impaired
Trauma, Risk for
Unilateral Neglect
Urinary Elimination, Impaired
Urinary Incontinence, Functional
Urinary Incontinence, Reflex
Urinary Incontinence, Risk for Urge

Urinary Incontinence, Stress
Urinary Incontinence, Total
Urinary Incontinence, Urge
Urinary Retention
Ventilation, Impaired Spontaneous
Ventilatory Weaning Response, Dysfunctional
Verbal Communication, Impaired
Violence, Risk for Other-Directed
Violence, Risk for Self-Directed
Walking, Impaired
Wandering
Weaning Response, Dysfunctional Ventilatory
Wheelchair Mobility, Impaired

Key Abbreviations and Acronyms Used in Healthcare*

AA	Alcoholics Anonymous		Ag	antigen
AFP	American Academy of Family Physicians		AGA	appropriate-for-gestational age
AALPN	American Association of Licensed Practical Nurses		AHA	American Hospital Association
			AHCPR	Agency for Health Care Policy and Research
AAMI	age-associated memory impairment		AI	adequate intake
AAP	American Academy of Pediatricians		AICD	automatic implantable cardioverter-defibrillator
AARP	American Association of Retired Persons		AIDS	acquired immunodeficiency syndrome
AB	abortion		AJN	American Journal of Nursing
Ab	antibody		AKA	above-the-knee amputation; also known as
ABCDE	Airway and cervical spine, breathing, circulation and bleeding, disability, expose and examine		ALL	acute lymphocytic leukemia
			ALS	amyotrophic lateral sclerosis
ABG	arterial blood gas(es)		ALT	aspartate aminotransferase (formerly SGOT)
ABP	acute bacterial prostatitis			
AC	Adriamycin (doxorubicin) and Cytoxan (cyclophosphamide)		AMA	against medical advice; American Medical Association
ACE	all cotton elastic; angiotensin-converting enzyme		AML	acute myelogenous leukemia
			ANA	American Nurses Association
ACIP	Advisory Committee on Immunization Practices		ANCC	American Nurses Credentialing Center
			ANP	atrial natriuretic peptide
ACLS	advanced cardiac life support		ANS	autonomic nervous system
ACOA	Adult Children of Alcoholics		AP	anterior-posterior (repair); anteroposterior; apical pulse; assault precautions (attack)
ACS	American Cancer Society; ambulatory care sensitive			
ACTH	adrenocorticotrophic hormone		APA	American Psychiatric Association
AD	advance directive		APGAR	A = appearance (color); P = pulse (heart rate); G = grimace or reflexes (irritability); A = activity (muscle tone); R = respiratory effort
ADA	American Diabetes Association			
ADAMHA	Alcohol, Drug Abuse, and Mental Health Administration			
ADC	AIDS dementia complex		APHA	American Public Health Association
ADDH	attention deficit disorder with hyperactivity		APIE	assessment, plan, intervention, evaluation
ADH	antidiuretic hormone		APTT	activated partial thromboplastin time
ADHD	attention deficit hyperactivity disorder		A-R	apical radial (pulse)
ADL	activities of daily living		ARC	American Red Cross
AEA	above-the-elbow amputation		ARDD	alcohol-related developmental disability
AEB	as evidenced by			
AED	automated external defibrillator		ARDS	adult respiratory distress syndrome
AFP	alpha-fetoprotein; α-fetoprotein		ARLD	alcohol-related liver disease
			ARND	alcohol-related neurodevelopmental disorder
			AROM	active range of motion; artificial rupture of the membranes

*Note: These are examples and may differ slightly from facility to facility.

ARRP	anatomic retropubic radical prostatectomy	C	Celsius; centigrade; kilocalorie
ART	Accredited Record Technician	C-2, C-3, etc.	refers to level of injury in the cervical section of the spinal cord
AS	sickle cell trait	Ca^{++}	calcium
ASA	acetylsalicylic acid (aspirin)	CABG	coronary artery bypass graft
ASD	atrial septal defect; autism spectrum disorders	$CaCl_2$	calcium chloride
		$CaCO_3$	calcium carbonate
ASI	addiciton severity index	CAD	coronary artery disease
ASO	antistreptolysin-O titer	CAF	Cytoxan (cyclophosphamide), Adriamycin (doxorubicin), fluorouracil
AST	aspartate aminotransferase		
ASU	ambulatory surgical unit		
ATF	Alcohol, Tobacco, and Firearms	CAPD	continuous ambulatory peritoneal dialysis
ATLS	advanced trauma life support		
ATN	acute tubular necrosis	$Ca_3[PO_4]_2$	calcium phosphate
ATP	adenosine triphosphate	CAT	computerized adaptive testing
AV	atrioventricular	CBC	complete blood count
AV node	atrioventricular node	CBE	charting by exception
AV valves	atrioventricular valves	CBP	chronic bacterial prostatitis
AVPU	alert, verbal, pain response, unresponsive	CC	chief complaint
		cc	cubic centimeter
AWOL	absent without leave	CCP	clinical care pathway
Ax	axillary	CCU	coronary care unit
		CCU/CICU	coronary care unit/coronary intensive care unit
BAL in oil	dimercaprol		
BBB	blood–brain barrier	CD	chemical dependency
BBP	blood-borne pathogen	CD4	helper T lymphocytes
BCG	bacillus Calmette-Guerin	CDC	Centers for Disease Control and Prevention
BCLS	basic cardiac life support		
BCP	birth control pill	CDU	chemical dependency unit, clinical decision unit
BE	barium enema x-ray		
BEA	below-the-elbow amputation	CEA	carcinoembryonic antigen; cultured epithelial autografts
BIDS	bedtime insulin and daytime sulfonylureas		
		CEH	continuing education hour
BKA	below-the-knee amputation	CEU	continuing education unit
BLL	blood lead level	CF	cystic fibrosis
BLS	basic (cardiac) life support	CHAP	Community Health Accreditation Program
BM	bowel movement		
BMI	body mass index	CHC	Community Health Center
BMT	bone marrow transplantation	CHD	coronary heart disease
BOA	born out of asepsis	CHF	congestive heart failure
BOH	Board of Health	CHHA	Certified Home Health Aide
BP	blood pressure	CHO	carbohydrates
BPAD	bipolar affective disorder	CIC	Crisis Intervention Center
BPD	bipolar disorder	CICU	coronary intensive care unit
BPH	benign prostatic hyperplasia	CK	creatine kinase
BPM	beats per minute	Cl	chloride
BPRS	Brief Psychiatric Rating Scale	CLL	chronic lymphocytic leukemia
BRAT	bananas, rice, applesauce, toast	CLTC	Citizens for Long-Term Care
BRM	biological response modifiers	CM	case/care manager
BRP	bathroom privileges	CMF	Cytoxan (cyclophosphamide), methotrexate, fluorouracil
BS	bowel sounds		
BSC	bedside commode	CMG	cystometrogram
BSE	breast self-examination	CML	chronic myelogenous leukemia
BUN	blood urea nitrogen	CMMS	Medicare and Medicaid Services

CMS	color, motion, sensitivity (circulation, mobility, sensation)	db	decibel
CMV	cytomegalovirus	DBP; dBP	diastolic blood pressure
CNM	Certified Nurse Midwife	D/C	discontinue
CNO	Community Nursing Organization	DCH	district court hold
CNS	central nervous system	DCT	distal convoluted tubule
CO	cardiac output	DDST	Denver Developmental Screening Test
CO_2	carbon dioxide	DEA	Drug Enforcement Agency
COA	children of alcoholics; coarctation of the aorta	DEP	Department of Environmental Protection
COAS	children of alcoholics	DERM	dermatology
COLD	chronic obstructive lung disease	DES	diethylstilbestrol
COPD	chronic obstructive pulmonary disease	DIC	disseminated intravascular coagulation
COPs	conditions of participation (Medicare requirements)	DIS	diagnostic interview schedule (for alcoholism)
COTA	Certified Occupational Therapy Assistant	DISCUS	Dyskinesia Identification System-Condensed User Scale
CP	cardiopulmonary; cerebral palsy	DJD	degenerative joint disease
CPAP	continuous positive airway pressure	DKA	diabetic ketoacidosis
CPD	cephalopelvic disproportion	DL	deciliter
CPK	creatine phosphokinase	DMAT	Disaster Medical Assistance Team
CPM	continuous passive motion	DMD	Duchenne's muscular dystrophy
CPR	cardiopulmonary resuscitation	DME	durable medical equipment
CPT	chest physiotherapy	DMSA	2, 3-dimercaptosuccinic acid
CQI	contiguous (or continuous) quality improvement	DNA	deoxyribonucleic acid
		DNH	do not hospitalize
CRH	corticotropin-releasing hormone	DNI	do not intubate
CRNA	Certified Registered Nurse Anesthetist	DNR	do not resuscitate
CRNH	Certified Registered Nurse—Hospice	DOA	Department of Agriculture
CRP	C-reactive protein	DOH	Department of Health
CRU	coronary rehabilitation unit	DOL	Department of Labor
Cryo	cryoprecipitate	DRF	drip rate factor
C & S	(blood) culture and sensitivity	DRG	diagnosis-related group
CS	cardiac sphincter; complete stroke	DRI	dietary reference intake
CSF	cerebrospinal fluid; colony-stimulating factors	DSM-IV	Diagnostic and Statistical Manual of Mental Disorders, Revision IV
CSR	Central Supply Room	DT	diphtheria and tetanus toxoids
CSS	Central Service Supply	DTAD	drain tube attachment device
CT	computed tomography	DTaP	diphtheria, tetanus, acellular pertussis
CUC	chronic ulcerative colitis	DTP	diphtheria and tetanus toxoids and pertussis vaccine
CVA	cerebrovascular accident		
CVP	central venous pressure	DTs	delirium tremens
CVS	chorionic villi sampling	DUI/DWI	driving while under the influence/driving while intoxicated
CXR	chest X-ray		
		DVR	Division of Vocational Rehabilitation
D & C	dilation and curettage	DVT	deep vein thrombosis
D/2NS5%	dextrose in half normal saline (0.45% NS)		
		EAR	estimated average requirement
D5NS5%	dextrose in normal saline (0.9% NS)	EC	emergency contraception
		ECF	extended care facility; extracellular fluid
D5W5%	dextrose in sterile water		
DAPE	data, assessment, plan, evaluation	ECG	electrocardiogram
DARE	data, action, response, education	ECT	Electroconvulsive therapy
DAT	diet as tolerated		

ED	Emergency Department; erectile dysfunction		5FU	5-flyorouracil
EDC	estimated date of confinement		FVD	fluid volume deficit
EDD	estimated date of delivery		FVE	fluid volume excess
EDTA	edetate calcium disodium		G	gauge
EEG	electroencephalogram; electroencephalography		G tube	gastrostomy tube
			G_6PD	glucose 6-phosphodehydrogenase
EGD	esophagogastroduodenoscopy		GABHS	group A beta-hemolytic streptococci
EHS	Employee Health Service		GCS	Glasgow Coma Scale
e-IPV	enhanced potency inactivated poliovirus vaccine		GDM	gestational diabetes mellitus
			GERD	gastroesophageal reflux disease
EKG	electrocardiogram		GERI	geriatrics
ELISA	enzyme-linked immunosorbent assay		GFR	glomerular filtration rate
EMB	ethambutol		GH	growth hormone
EMG	electromyogram		GHIH	growth hormone-inhibiting hormone
EMS	Emergency Medical Services		GHRH	growth hormone-releasing hormone
EMT	Emergency Medical Technician		GI	gastrointestinal
ENG	electronystagmography		GnRH	gonadotropin-releasing hormone
EP	escape (elopement) precaution		GRH	growth hormone-releasing hormone
EPA	Environmental Protection Agency		GTT	glucose tolerance test
EPO	erythropoietin		G-tube	gastrostomy tube
EPS	electrophysiology study		GU	genitourinary
EPSE	extrapyramidal side effects		GYN	gynecology
ERCP	endoscopic retrograde cholangiopancreatography		H^+	hydrogen ion
ERG	electroretinogram		H_2CO_3	carbonic acid
ERT	estrogen replacement therapy		H_2O	water
ERV	expiratory reserve volume		$H_2PO_4^-$	Phosphate
ESR	erythrocyte sedimentation rate		HAS	Health Services Administration
ESRD	end-stage renal disease		HAV	hepatitis A virus
ESWL	extracorporeal shockwave lithotripsy		HAZMAT	hazardous materials
ET	enterostomal therapist		Hb	hemoglobin
ETOH	ethanol (alcohol)		$Hb\ A_{1c}$	glycosylated hemoglobin
ETOH W/D	alcohol withdrawal		HBD	hydroxybutyric dehydrogenase
			HBO	hyperbaric oxygenation
F	Fahrenheit		HBV	hepatitis B virus
FADL	functional activities of daily living		HCA	Health Care Assistant
FAM	fertility awareness method		HCFA	Health Care Financing Association (payer source)
FAS	fetal alcohol syndrome			
FBP	fetal biophysical profile		HCG	human chorionic gonadotropin
FBS	fasting blood sugar (fasting blood glucose)		HCl	hydrochloric acid
			HCO_3^-	bicarbonate
FDA	Food and Drug Administration		Hct	hematocrit
Fe^{++}	iron		HCTZ	hydrochlorothiazide
FES	functional electrical stimulation		HCV	hepatitis C virus
FFP	fresh frozen plasma		HD	Hodgkin's disease; Huntington's disease
FHC	Family Health Center			
FHR	fetal heart rate		HDL	high-density lipoprotein
FHT	fetal heart tones		HDV	hepatitis D virus
FPG	fasting plasma glucose		HEV	hepatitis E virus
FQHC	federally qualified healthcare		HFCS	high-fructose corn syrup
FRC	functional residual capacity		H flu	Haemophilus influenzae
FRV	functional residue volume		Hgb	hemoglobin
FSH	follicle-stimulating hormone		HGF	hematopoietic factor
FTT	failure to thrive		HGV	hepatitis G virus

HHA	Home Health Aide		InFeD	iron dextran
HHRG	Home Health Resource Group		INH	isoniazid
HHS	Department of Health and Human Services		I & O	intake and output
HI	homicidal ideation		IOL	intraocular lens
Hib	Haemophilus influenzae type-B conjugate vaccine		IOL implant	intraocular lens implant
HICPAC	Hospital Infection Control Practices Advisory Committee		IOP	intraocular pressure
			IPPB	intermittent positive pressure breathing
HIS	Indian Health Service		IQ	intelligence quotient
HIV	human immunodeficiency virus		IR	infrared (rays)
HIV-RNA	viral load of HIV		IRV	inspiratory reserve volume
HMO	health maintenance organization		ITP	idiopathic thrombocytopenic purpura
HNP	herniated nucleus pulposus		IUD	intrauterine device
HOSA	Health Occupations Students of America		IV	intravenous
			IVC	inferior vena cava
hPL	human placental lactogen		IVD	intervertebral disk disease
HPO_4^{--}	phosphate		IVF	in vitro fertilization
2hPP	2-hour post-prandial		IVIG	intravenous immune globulin
HPV	human papilloma virus		IVP	intravenous pyelogram
HR	heart rate		IVPB	intravenous piggyback
HRT	hormone replacement therapy			
HS	hour of sleep		J tube	jejunostomy tube
HSV-1	herpes simplex virus type 1		JCAHO	Joint Commission on Accreditation of Healthcare Organizations
HSV-2	herpes simplex virus type 2			
HTN	hypertension		JG	juxtaglomerular
HUS	hemolytic uremic syndrome		JGA	juxtaglomerular apparatus
			JP	Jackson-Pratt (drain)
IADL	instrumental activities of daily living		JRA	juvenile rheumatoid arthritis
IBD	inflammatory bowel disease			
IBS	irritable bowel syndrome		K^+	potassium
IBW	ideal body weight		Kcal	kilocalorie
IC	interstitial cystitis; inspiratory capacity		KCl	potassium chloride
			KOH	potassium hydroxide
ICD	implantable cardioverter–defibrillator		KUB	kidney, ureter, and bladder x-ray
ICF	intermediate care facility			
ICN	International Council of Nurses		L-1, L-2, etc.	refers to level of injury in the lumbar area of the spinal cord
ICP	increased intercranial pressure			
ICP	intracranial pressure		LAD	left anterior descending
ICSH	interstitial cell-stimulating hormone		LASIK	laser-assisted in situ keratomileusis
ICU	intensive care unit		LATCH	L = latch; A = audible swallowing; T = type of nipple; C = comfort (breast/nipple); H = hold (positioning)
ID	identification			
IDDM	insulin-dependent diabetes mellitus			
IDG	interdisciplinary group			
IDT	interdisciplinary team		LBW	low birth weight
IFG	impaired fasting glucose		LCA	left coronary artery
IFN	interferon		LCX	left circumflex
Ig	immunoglobulin(s)		LDH	lactic dehydrogenase
IgE	immunoglobulin E		LDL	low-density lipoprotein
IgG	immunoglobulin G (gamma globulin)		LDRP	labor/delivery/recovery/postpartum room
IGH	impaired glucose homeostasis			
IGT	impaired glucose tolerance		LEEP	loop electrosurgical excision procedure
II	intellectual impairment		LEP	laparoscopic extraperitoneal approach
IICP	increased intracranial pressure		LES	lower esophageal sphincter
IL	interleukin		LFT	liver function tests
			LGA	large for gestational age

LH	leuteinizing hormone	MMR	measles, mumps, and rubella
LLQ	left lower quadrant	MOM	milk of magnesia
LMCA	left main coronary artery	MPD	multiple personality disorder
L/min	liters per minute	MRI	magnetic resonance imaging
LMP	last menstrual period	MRSA	Methicillin-resistant Staphylococcus
LNMP	last normal menstrual period		aureus
LOC	level of consciousness	MS	morphine sulfate; multiple sclerosis
LP	lumbar puncture	MSAFP	maternal serum alpha-fetoprotein
LPM	liters per minute		(test)
LPN	Licensed Practical Nurse	MSDS	Material Safety Data Sheet
LQR	locked quiet room	MSH	melanocyte-stimulating hormone
LSD	lysergic acid diethylamide	MSW	Medical Social Worker
LSR	locked seclusion room	MUA	medically underserved areas
Ls ratio	lecithin/sphingomyelin ratio	MVA	motor vehicle accident
LT	leukotriene		
LTB	laryngotracheobronchitis	NA	Narcotics Anonymous
LTC	long-term care	Na+	sodium
LUQ	left upper quadrant	Na₂SO₄	sodium sulfate
LVN	Licensed Vocational Nurse	NACHC	National Association of Community
			Health Centers
MABP	mean arterial blood pressure	NaCl	sodium chloride
MAC	mycobacterium avium complex	NAHC	National Association for Home Care
MADD	Mothers Against Drunk Driving	NAHCC	National Association of Health Care
MAP	mean arterial pressure		Centers
MAR	Medication Administration Record	NANDA	North American Nursing Diagnosis
MAST	military antishock trousers		Association
MCHB	Maternal Child Health Bureau	NaOH	sodium hydroxide
MD	muscular dystrophy	NAPNES	National Association of Practical
MDA/	methylenedioxyamphetamine/		Nurse Education and Services
MDMA	methylenedioxymethamphetamine	NCHS	National Center for Health Statistics
	("ecstasy")	NCI	National Cancer Institute
MDD	major depressive disorder	NCLEX	National Council Licensure
MDI	metered dose inhaler		Examination
MDS	minimum data set	NCLEX-PN	National Council Licensure
mEq	milliequivalent		Examination for Practical Nurses
mEq/L	milliequivalents per liter	NCLEX-RN	National Council Licensure
Mg	magnesium		Examination for Registered Nurses
MG	myasthenia gravis	NCP	nursing care plan
mg/dL	milligrams per deciliter	NCSBN	National Council of State Boards of
Mg++	magnesium		Nursing
MgSO₄	magnesium sulfate	NEC	necrotizing enterocolitis
MH	mental health	NEURO	neurology
MHU	mental health unit	NF	National Formulary
MI	mental illness; myocardial infarction	NFLPN	National Federation of Licensed
MI-CD	mentally ill and chemically dependant		Practical Nurses
MICU	medical intensive care unit	NG	nasogastric
MI & D	mentally ill and dangerous	NG tube	nasogastric tube
MIF	melanocyte-inhibiting	NHIC	National Health Information Center
MIS	Management Information	NHL	non-Hodgkin's lymphoma
	Services/Systems	NHO	National Hospice Organization
MJ	marijuana ("weed")	NHP	Nursing Home Placement
mL	milliliter	NHPCO	National Hospice and Palliative Care
MMI	methimazole		Organization
MMPI	Minnesota Multiphasic Personality	NICU	neonatal intensive care unit
	Inventory		

NIDDM	non-insulin-dependent diabetes mellitus		OU	both eyes (oculi unitas)
NIH	National Institutes of Health		P	phosphorous
NINR	National Institute of Nursing Research		PA	Physician Assistant
NIOSH	National Institute of Occupational Safety and Health		PACE	Pre-Admission and Classification Examination
NLN	National League for Nursing		paCO$_2$	carbon dioxide content of arterial blood
NMR	nuclear magnetic resonance		PACU	postanesthesia care unit
NMS	neuroleptic malignant syndrome		paO$_2$	oxygen content of arterial blood
NOS	not otherwise specified		Pap test	Papanicolaou test (smear)
NP	Nurse Practitioner		PAR	postanesthesia recovery (room)
NPO	nothing by mouth		PBI	protein-bound iodine
NPT	nocturnal penile tumescence		PBSC	peripheral blood stem cell
NRM	non-rebreathing mask		PCA	patient-controlled analgesia; personal care attendant
NS	normal saline (0.9% sodium chloride)			
NSAID	nonsteroidal anti-inflammatory drug		PCM	protein-calorie malnutrition
NSC	National Safety Council		PCN	penicillin
NST	nonstress test		pCO$_2$	carbon dioxide content of arterial blood
NTG	nitroglycerine		PCP	phencyclidine HCl ("angel dust"); *Pneumocystis carinii* pneumonia; primary care provider
O$_2$	oxygen			
O$_2$Sat	percent oxygen saturation			
OA	osteoarthritis		PCT	proximal convoluted tubule
OASIS	Outcome and Assessment Information Set		PDA	patent ductus arteriosus; posterior descending artery
OB	obstetrics		PDR	Physician's Desk Reference
OBD	organic brain disorder		PE (tube)	polyethylene (tube)
OB/GYN	obstetrician/gynecologist		PEDS	pediatrics
OBRA	Omnibus Budget Reconciliation Act		PEG	percutaneous endoscopic gastrostomy
OBS	organic brain syndrome		PEP	postexposure prophylaxis
OBT	over-bed table		PERRLA+C	pupils equal, round, react to light, accommodation OK and coordinated
OCD	obsessive compulsive disorder			
OCT	oxytocin challenge test			
OD	right eye (oculus dexter); overdose		PET	position emission tomography scan
OFC	occipital-frontal circumference		PFT	pulmonary function test
OH$^-$	hydroxyl ion		pH	potential of hydrogen or power of hydrogen (hydrogen ion concentration)
OMH	Office for Migrant Health			
ONS	Oncology Nursing Society			
OOB	out of bed		PIA	prolonged infantile apnea
OP	occiput posterior, direct		PIC	peripheral indwelling catheter
O & P	ova (eggs) and parasites		PIC line	peripheral indwelling catheter
OPD	Outpatient Department		PICC	peripherally inserted central catheter
OPHS	Office of Public Health and Science		PICU	pediatric intensive care unit
OPV	(live) oral poliovirus vaccine		PID	pelvic inflammatory disease
OR	operating room		PIE	plan, intervention, evaluation
ORIF	open reduction and internal fixation		PIH	pregnancy-induced hypertension; prolactin-inhibiting
ORS	oral rehydration solution			
ORTHO	orthopedics		PKR	photorefractive keratotomy
OS	left eye (oculus sinister)		PKU	phenylketonuria
OSHA	Occupational Safety and Health Administration		PMI	point of maximal impulse
			PMP	previous menstrual period
OT	occupational therapy		PM&R	physical medicine and rehabilitation
OTC	over the counter		PMS	premenstrual syndrome
OTR	Occupational Therapist, Registered		PNS	peripheral nervous system
			PO	by mouth (per os)

pO_2	oxygen content of arterial blood
POC	plan of care
POS	point of service
PPD	purified protein derivative
PPE	personal protective equipment
PPF	plasma protein fraction
PPG	postprandial glucose
PPIP	put prevention into practice
PPN	peripheral parenteral nutrition
PPO	preferred provider organization
PPROM	premature rupture of the membranes
PPS	prospective payment system
PRH	prolactin-releasing hormone
PRL	prolactin
PRM	partial-rebreathing mask
PRN	as needed
PROM	passive range of motion; premature rupture of membranes
PR/R	per rectum/rectal
PSA	prostate-specific antigen
PSDA	Patient Self-Determination Act
psi	per square inch
PSV	pressure support ventilation
PSYCH	psychiatry
PT	physical therapy; prothrombin time
PTA	Physical Therapist Assistant
PTCA	percutaneous transluminal coronary angioplasty
PTH	parathormone; parathyroid hormone
PTL	preterm labor
PTSD	post-traumatic stress disorder
PTT	partial thromboplastin time
PTU	propylthiouracil
PUBS	percutaneous umbilical blood sampling
PUS	prostate ultrasound
PVC	premature ventricular contraction
PZA	pyrazinamide
QA	quality assurance
QI	quality improvement
RA	rheumatoid arthritis
RAA	renin-angiotensin-aldosterone
RACE	rescue, alarm, confine, extinguish
RAI	radioactive iodine
RAIU	radioactive iodine uptake
RAP	resident assessment protocol
RBC	red blood cell
RCA	right coronary artery
RDA	recommended dietary allowance
RDS	respiratory distress syndrome
REE	resting energy expenditure
REHAB	rehabilitation unit
REM	rapid eye movement

RET/REBT	Rational Emotive (Behavior) Therapy
RF	rheumatoid factor
RGP	rigid gas-permeable plastic
Rh+	Rh positive
Rh-	Rh negative
RhoGAM®	Rh immune globulin
RICE	rest, ice, compression, elevation
RIE	recorded in error
RIND	reversible ischemic neurologic deficit
RK	radial keratotomy
RLQ	right lower quadrant
RMP	rifampin
RN	Registered Nurse
RNA	ribonucleic acid
ROI	release of information
ROM	range of motion
ROP	retinopathy of prematurity; right occiput posterior
RP	retinitis pigmentosa
RPh	Registered Pharmacist
RPT	Registered Physical Therapist
RR	recovery room
RRA	Registered Record Administrator
RSV	respiratory syncytial virus
RT	respiratory therapy
R/T	related to
RUG	resource utilization group
RUQ	right upper quadrant
RV	residual volume
S_1	the first heart sound
S_2	the second heart sound
S/A	suicide attempt
SA node	sinoatrial node or sinus node
SBE	subacute bacterial endocarditis
SBFT	small bowel follow-through x-ray
SBP; sBP	systolic blood pressure
SDSU	same day surgery unit
Sed rate	erythrocyte sedimentation rate
S/G	suicide gesture
SGA	small for gestational age
SGOT	serum glutamic oxaloacetic transaminase
SI units	International System of Units (or Systeme International d'Unites)
SI	suicidal ideation
SIADH	syndrome of inappropriate antidiuretic hormone
SIB	self-injurious behavior
SICU	surgical intensive care unit
SIDS	sudden infant death syndrome
SIE	stroke in evolution
SIMV	synchronized intermittent mandatory ventilation

SIRES	stabilize, identify toxin, reverse effect, eliminate toxin, support		TED	thromboembolitic disease
SL	sublingual		TEE	transesophageal echocardiography
SLD	specific learning disabilities		TENS	transcutaneous electrical nerve stimulation
SLE	systemic lupus erythematosus		TFT	thyroid function test
S/M	sadomasochism		TGV	transposition of the great vessels
SMBG	self-monitoring of blood glucose		THA	total hip arthroplasty
SNF	skilled nursing facility		THC	tetrahydrocannabinol; cannabis (marijuana and related drugs)
SNS	sympathetic nervous system			
SO	significant other		T-hold	transportation hold (police)
SO_4^{--}	sulfate		TIA	transient ischemic attack
SOAP	subjective, objective, assessment, plan		TICU	trauma intensive care unit
			Title XIX	Medicaid Section of the Social Security Act
SOAPIER	subjective, objective, assessment, plan, intervention, evaluation, response		Title XVIII	Medicare Section of the Social Security Act
SOB	short of breath		Title XXII	Source of COPs
SOBOE	short of breath on exertion		TKA	total knee arthroplasty
SP	suprapubic (catheter)		TLC	total lung capacity
SP/GP	suicide precautions/general precautions		TLSO	thoracolumbosacral orthosis
			Tm	transport maximum
SPF	sun protective factor		TMJ	temporomandibular joint
SRO	single room occupancy		TMR	transmyocardial revascularization
SROM	spontaneous rupture of the membranes		TO	telephone order
			TOF	tetralogy of Fallot
SSA	Social Security Administration		TORCH	toxoplasmosis, other, rubella, cytomegalovirus, herpes simplex
SSDI	Social Security Disability Insurance			
SSE	soapsuds enema		t-PA	tissue plasminogen activator
START	simple triage and rapid treatment		TPA	total parenteral alimentation
STAT	at once, immediately		TPN	total parenteral nutrition
STD	sexually transmitted disease		TPR	temperature, pulse and respiration
STH	somatotropic hormone; somatotropin		TR	therapeutic recreation
			TS	Tourette's syndrome
STI	sexually transmitted infection		TSE	testicular self-examination
STP	sodium thiopental (Pentothal)		TSH	thyroid-stimulating hormone
SV	stroke volume		TSLO	thoracic-lumbar-sacral orthosis
SVC	superior vena cava		TSS	toxic shock syndrome
SVE	sterile vaginal examination		TURBT	transurethral resection of a bladder tumor
SVR	systemic vascular resistance			
SX P	sexual precautions		TURP	transurethral resection of the prostate
SZ P	seizure precautions			
			TV	tidal volume
T-1, T-2, etc.	refers to level of injury in the thoracic area of the spinal cord		TWE	tap water enema
			T & X	type and crossmatch
T^3	triiodothyronine			
T^4	thyroxine		U-100	100 units per milliliter
T&A	tonsillectomy and adenoidectomy		UA	urinalysis
TAC	time, amount, character		UAP	unlicensed assistive personnel
TB	tuberculosis		UL	tolerance upper intake level
TBI	traumatic brain injury		UN	United Nations
TBW	total body water		UNICEF	United Nations Children's Fund
TCDB	turning, coughing, deep breathing		UNOS	United Network of Organ Sharing
TCN	tetracycline		UPP	urethral pressure profile
TD	tardive dyskinesia		UPT	urine pregnancy test

URI	upper respiratory infection		VMA	vanillylmandelic acid
UROL	urology		VNA	Visiting Nurse Association
US	ultrasound		VO	verbal order
USD	United States Dispensatory		Vol	voluntarily admitted
USDA	United States Department of Agriculture		VRE	vancomycin-resistant enterococci
USDHHS	United States Department of Health and Human Services		V & S	volume and specific gravity (urine)
			VSD	ventricular septal defect
USP	United States Pharmacopeia			
USPHS	United States Public Health Service		WA	while awake
UTI	urinary tract infection		WBC	white blood cell
UTox	urine toxicity screen (for drugs)		W/C	wheelchair
UV	ultraviolet (rays)		W/D	withdrawal
			WHO	World Health Organization
			WIC	women, infants and children
VC	vital capacity		WISC-R	Wechsler Intelligence Scale for Children—Revised
VCUG	voiding cystourethrogram			
VLBW	very low birth weight		WKS	Wernicke–Korsakoff syndrome
			WNL	within normal limits

PROGRAM LICENSE AGREEMENT

Read carefully the following terms and conditions before using the Software. Use of the Software indicates you and, if applicable, your Institution's acceptance of the terms and conditions of this License Agreement. If you do not agree with the terms and conditions, you should promptly return this package to the place you purchased it and your payment will be refunded.

Definitions

As used herein, the following terms shall have the following meanings:

"Software" means the software program contained on the diskette(s) or CD-ROM or preloaded on a workstation and the user documentation, which includes all accompanying printed material.

"Institution" means a nursing or professional school, a single academic organization that does not provide patient care and is located in a single city and has one geographic location/address.

"Geographic location" means a facility at a specific location; geographic locations do not provide for satellite or remote locations that are considered a separate facility.

"Facility" means a health care facility at a specific location that provides patient care and is located in a single city and has one geographic location/address.

"Publisher" means Lippincott Williams & Wilkins, Inc., with its principal office in Philadelphia, Pennsylvania.

"Developer" means the company responsible for developing the software as noted on the product.

License

You are hereby granted a nonexclusive license to use the Software in the United States. This license is not transferable and does not authorize resale or sublicensing without the written approval or an authorized officer of Publisher.

The Publisher retains all rights and title to all copyrights, patents, trademarks, trade secrets, and other proprietary rights in the Software. You may not remove or obscure the copyright notices in or on the Software. You agree to use reasonable efforts to protect the Software from unauthorized use, reproduction, distribution or publication.

Single-User license

If you purchased this Software program at the Single-User License price or a discount of that price, you may use this program on one single-user computer. You may not use the Software in a time-sharing environment or otherwise to provide multiple, simultaneous access. You may not provide or permit access to this program to anyone other than yourself.

Institutional/Facility license

If you purchased the Software at the Institutional or Facility License Price or at a discount of that price, you have purchased the Software for use within your Institution/Facility on a single workstation/computer. You may not provide copies of or remote access to the Software. You may not modify or translate the program or related documentation. You agree to instruct the individuals in your Institution/Facility who will have access to the Software to abide by the terms of this License Agreement. If you or any member of your Institution fail to comply with any of the terms of this License Agreement, this license shall terminate automatically.

Network license

If you purchased the Software at the Network License Price, you may copy the Software for use within your Institution/Facility on an unlimited number of computers within one geographic location/address. You may not provide remote access to the Software over a value-added network or otherwise. You may not provide copies of or remote access to the Software to individuals or entities who are not members of your Institution/Facility. You may not modify or translate the program or related documentation. You agree to instruct the individuals in your Institution/Facility who will have access to the Software to abide by the terms of this License Agreement. If you or any member of your Institution/Facility fail to comply with any of the terms of this License Agreement, this license shall terminate automatically.

Limited warranty

The Publisher warrants that the media on which the Software is furnished shall be free from defects in materials and workmanship under normal use for a period of 90 days from the date of delivery to you, as evidenced by your receipt of purchase.

The Software is sold on a 30-day trial basis. If, for whatever reason, you decide not to keep the software, you may return it for a full refund within 30 days of the invoice date or purchase, as evidenced by your receipt of purchase by returning all parts of the Software and packaging in saleable condition with the original invoice, to the place you purchased it. If the Software is not returned in such condition, you will not be entitled to a refund. When returning the Software, we suggest that you insure all packages for their retail value and mail them by a traceable method.

The Software is a computer assisted instruction (CAI) program that is not intended to provide medical consultation regarding the diagnosis or treatment of any specific patient.

The Software is provided without warranty of any kind, either expressed or implied, including but not limited to any implied warranty of fitness for a particular purpose of merchantability. Neither Publisher nor Developer warrants that the Software will satisfy your requirements or that the Software is free of program or content errors. Neither Publisher nor Developer warrants, guarantees, or makes any representation regarding the use of the Software in terms of accuracy, reliability or completeness, and you rely on the content of the programs solely at your own risk.

The Publisher is not responsible (as a matter of products liability, negligence or otherwise) for any injury resulting from any material contained herein. This Software contains information relating to general principles of patient care that should not be construed as specific instructions for individual patients. Manufacturers' product information and package inserts should be reviewed for current information, including contraindications, dosages and precautions.

Some states do not allow the exclusion of implied warranties, so the above exclusion may not apply to you. This warranty gives you specific legal rights and you may also have other rights that vary from state to state.

Limitation of remedies

The entire liability of Publisher and Developer and your exclusive remedy shall be: (1) the replacement of any CD which does not meet the limited warranty stated above which is returned to the place you purchased it with your purchase receipt; or (2) if the Publisher or the wholesaler or retailer from whom you purchased the Software is unable to deliver a replacement CD free from defects in material and workmanship, you may terminate this License Agreement by returning the CD, and your money will be refunded.

In no event will Publisher or Developer be liable for any damages, including any damages for personal injury, lost profits, lost savings or other incidental or consequential damages arising out of the use or inability to use the Software or any error or defect in the Software, whether in the database or in the programming, even if the Publisher, Developer, or an authorized wholesaler or retailer has been advised of the possibility of such damage.

Some states do not allow the limitation or exclusion of liability for incidental or consequential damages. The above limitations and exclusions may not apply to you.

General

This License Agreement shall be governed by the laws of the State of Pennsylvania without reference to the conflict of laws provisions thereof, and may only be modified in a written statement signed by an authorized officer of the Publisher. By opening and using the Software, you acknowledge that you have read this License Agreement, understand it, and agree to be bound by its terms and conditions. You further agree that it is a complete and exclusive statement of the agreement between the Institution/Facility and the Publisher, which supersedes any proposal or prior agreement, oral or written, and any other communication between you and Publisher or Developer relative to the subject matter of the License Agreement.

Note

Attach a paid invoice to the License Agreement as proof of purchase.

Testbank CD-ROM to Accompany
Rosdahl & Kowalski's Textbook of Basic Nursing, Eighth Edition

INSTALLATION INSTRUCTIONS

Insert the CD into the CD-ROM drive on your PC.

There are several ways to view the contents of the CD:

- Open the Start menu, go to Programs, then go to Windows Explorer. Windows Explorer will open, and you will see the icon for the CD-ROM drive on the left side of the screen. Click on the icon and the contents of the CD will appear on the right side of the screen.
- On your desktop, double-click on the "My Computer" icon. Then double-click on the icon for the CD-ROM drive. A new window will pop up with the contents of the CD.
- Hold down the Window key on your keyboard and tap the "E" key. Windows Explorer will open, and the icon for the CD-ROM drive will be on the left side of the screen. Click on the icon and the contents of the CD will appear on the right side of the screen.

Double click on any folder to view the files inside the folder.

Double click on any file to view its content.

You will need a word-processing program (e.g., MS Word or WordPerfect) to open the files on this CD.

Angeles College
3440 Wilshire Blvd., Suite 310
Los Angeles, CA 90010
Tel. (213) 487-2211